What oth

"Nothing unsettles an athlete   ind few injuries are more common to endurance athletes than plantar fasciitis. Now Patrick Hafner offers hope, and relief, with a clearly stated plan for recovery and prevention."

Joe Henderson, co-author of *Running Injury-Free*

"I recommend Injury Afoot for anyone who has feet. It's a must-read resource, chockfull of easy-to-follow tips to help alleviate a flare up of plantar fasciitis and then keep it from coming back."

Liz Neporent, president of Wellness 360 (w360.com) and author of *Weight Training for Dummies*.

"We meet several folks a day who experience these symptoms. My response reflects what you teach in the book, and that is to do as much non-interventional treatment as you can, as soon as you can, because you never know for sure what will be the healing trigger appropriate for you. Sometimes it just takes a 'full frontal assault' of everything you can bring to bear on it. You have provided for us the best answer for our many suffering customers. 'Here are shoes that fit and work for you. Here's a good footbed. Here are some other items that could help, but most of all here is a great book!'"

Steve Roguski, owner, Fairhaven Runners & Walkers, www.FairhavenRunners.com

Injury Afoot

30 Things You Can Do to Relieve Heel Pain and Speed Healing of Plantar Fasciitis

Patrick Hafner

Birchbark Publishing

Publisher's Cataloging in Publication

Hafner, Patrick

Injury afoot: 30 things you can do to relieve heel pain and speed healing of plantar fasciitis / Patrick Hafner

p.   cm.

Includes index.

ISBN-13: 978-0-9801724-5-4

1. Foot injury -- rehabilitation.   I. Title

617.1027

Library of Congress Control Number: 2008903993

To Béatrice: wouldn't have been possible without you.

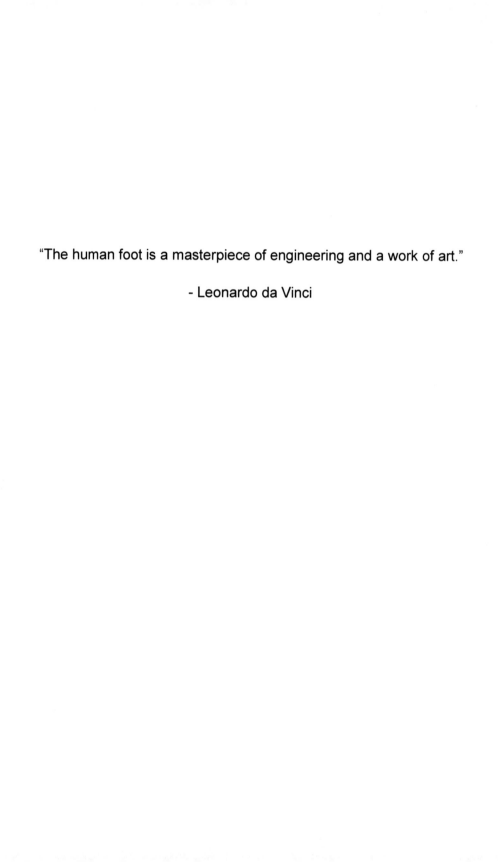

"The human foot is a masterpiece of engineering and a work of art."

- Leonardo da Vinci

Contents

Disclaimer

Consult with your physician before you begin to participate in any workout or exercise program, including exercises in this book. I'm not a medical professional and do not claim to be. I've used all the activities and advice which I've listed within, and the described routine helped my feet heal from plantar fasciitis. I have confidence in the enclosed advice and believe it will help you as it did me. However, as required in books of this type, I must state that using the guidelines included in the following pages is done at your own risk.

Preface

The collapse of my exercise program snuck up on me like a shark rising in silence from the depths. Then it sunk its teeth into my feet. And shook.

At the time, I was no stranger to the rigors of regular exercise. I had been through just about all the stresses and strains possible from strenuous workouts, and had kept at it for many years. I had just finished my sixth season as a recreational but serious runner, training for and running races year-round. During that time, I had completed numerous 5Ks and 10Ks, four 10-mile races, and three half marathons. I wasn't really born with the ideal body type of a long distance runner, with a heavier, stockier frame than that of many running competitors. As a rhinoceros running amongst gazelles, my lower body took a significant beating. I endured frequent shin splints, a tenderized lower back, pummeled hamstring muscles, and pulverized calves over the course of most races. Yet despite the beatings, my body would soon recover after a bit of rest, and I'd be back out running in no time.

Before I became serious about running, I was a hardcore wrestler and judo competitor for 15 years. Between practice and tournaments, I was slammed, wrenched, and twisted into a pretzel regularly. Aches and pains cropped up in my knees, shoulders, neck, and just about every other place. But similar to my running experience, I conquered each injury with a little rest, a little ice, and a little time. I was never incapacitated to any great extent, and never experienced a long layoff due to injury.

In addition, during the 20 years plus spent between running and wrestling sports, I never encountered a problem with my feet. Not once. And every other athletic-related setback was so temporary I'd soon forget I had even experienced it. I knew I wasn't indestructible, but after rounding the 40-year mark, and still grinding away with a rigorous exercise regimen, I began to see myself as a bit unstoppable. One of those few who could just keep going and going. Heck, I didn't even need to stretch.

Then plantar fasciitis twirled into my life like a buzz saw, severing that illusion.

It started out as a hint of discomfort. Just an insignificant intruder down in the back of my shoe. At first, I ignored it and continued on with my activities. In fact, as I ran, the slight pain disappeared, and I could then complete the course. Sure, the pain would recur, especially first thing in the morning, but I unknowingly assumed it was another short term battle scar. And I could just run it off. The pain transformed from slight to sharp, at times intense enough to make me limp. I'd just run a little faster. A little longer. Problem solved. Until the pain returned that evening, and even more so the next morning. I continued to push through it, and waited for the injury, whatever it was, to heal itself.

This cycle continued until I could no longer run without excessive discomfort. I was lucky to be able to go for a walk without pain. At that point, one or both feet would fire up with alarming pain upon my first few steps out of bed. This began to occur most mornings. Sometimes it was bad enough that I would need to steady myself on the dresser or a piece of furniture to avoid the piercing feeling. As the morning progressed, my feet would loosen up and walking became possible. Most of the discomfort would subside for the time being. However, the waves of pain would generally resume in the evening.

The situation became unpredictable. The soreness remained for a while, but within a couple of weeks it started to fade. Bingo, I'm healed. Great, I'm going running. And out I went, and ran myself right back to square one. The return of the swelling and painful flare-ups was worse than ever. I had mistakenly jumped back in too soon, and running became out of the question. The discomfort developed into the sensation of a steak knife sticking into my heel. I even stopped walking to let my feet rest. Give them a break for two or three weeks, I figured.

Four months after my exercise regimen was derailed, the plantar fasciitis remained. It became clear to me this was no ordinary injury. No more running, no more rigorous hikes. Long walks were hazardous. I could barely stroll through the house without limping. Standing in place in a grocery store became painful.

Terror started to mount. What had I done to myself? I began to suspect the worst. Was I now crippled? As far as I could remember, all I did was run a lot, walk a little, and go on some hikes. Aren't those things supposed to be good for you?

After some quick research, I verified that these grueling symptoms were in fact classic signs of plantar fasciitis, a condition I had heard of now and then but hadn't thought about much. Some sources even referred to it as the "dreaded plantar fasciitis." Couldn't have said it better myself.

Now desperate, I scrambled to find more information on treating plantar fasciitis. The condition is mainly remedied with home treatment, it turned out. Surgery is rarely recommended, and often not helpful even if it is used as a solution. I had found a few suggestions on how to relieve plantar fasciitis, and put them into practice. But these brief bits of advice were only pieces of the puzzle. I needed more to whip this thing.

So I became a hunter-gatherer of information. As I began an exhaustive search for answers, I uncovered snippets of advice here and there. Some books had only a single page covering plantar fasciitis, and some reputable exercise magazines contained a single short article, often less than a page. Some websites presented a checklist telling *what* to do, but not many details on *how* to do those things. I rarely came across bad advice. It was all valuable, but on the other hand, it was too brief. Avoid this, stretch that, you're healed, on to the next subject.

But that wasn't what I was realizing; it wasn't what I was living. The dilemma of healing a case of plantar fasciitis turned out to be tricky and complex. I was reminded of this with each wince in the morning upon my first steps out of bed. Reminded of it with each rest break I was forced to take after just a few blocks of walking. Or with each stop to adjust my shoes and stretch just to complete my walk. I was reminded of this for months, as time rolled by and my feet didn't heal.

There's not one simple remedy for plantar fasciitis. And there's not just one cause of it, and not just one category of athlete, exerciser, worker, or walker who can acquire it. In my opinion, the intricacies of treating plantar fasciitis warranted more than just one page in a book or a short article. And this was further evidenced by the range of treatment information I uncovered: different sources stated completely different suggestions. The sources didn't contradict each other, really. They simply gave different directions to heal the same condition. And this illustrates a couple of things: 1) the severity of plantar fasciitis can vary greatly, and 2) the vast array of body types, fitness levels, and foot characteristics respond in unpredictable ways to a given treatment. Everyone is unique. The specifics of each person's injury can be unique also, and what works for one person may not be right for another. Or it may not be enough. For plantar fasciitis rehab, a lot of information and a lot of possible recovery actions are a good thing.

I proceeded to locate and harness every bit of plantar fasciitis treatment info I could find and consolidate all of it: to gather the facts, make sense of them, and work out a system to get my feet healthy again. Using the findings and advice of researchers, elite athletes, and medical professionals, I devised my own recuperation plan. I even found out a few things by experimentation that spared me some pain and helped me avoid reinjury. I added these items to the plan as I went.

Did the recuperation plan work? Well, at the most severe point in my plantar fasciitis trauma, I could barely walk five blocks. Six months after committing to the plan, I ran all-out in the Portland Marathon's 5-mile race. In the days following the race, I experienced no additional discomfort in my feet, despite the grueling run (the rest of my body hurt, but I digress!). And in the next few months, I ran several more races and hiked and walked countless miles. My feet continue to hold out and withstand such rigors to this day.

Do I have some magic formula that cures the pain in your feet instantly? Absolutely not. I don't think one exists. But I took information gathered over months and compiled it together into one central source. Everything I could find regarding conservative, non-interventional plantar fasciitis therapy has been included in this book. And I personally used each and every action item listed. I had motivation, believe me. I hated being injured. I wanted to get back into the action. I wanted to walk normally again. I wanted to be able to stand in place without pain. If you're suffering from plantar fasciitis, however mild or severe, you know what I mean.

This book assumes you have begun to experience the symptoms of plantar fasciitis. Tender arches. Pain in your heel, perhaps at the very back of it or where it meets the arch. Maybe in both of these spots, and at the outside edge of your foot as well. And it's at its worst first thing in the morning, lets up a bit as the day goes on, then returns again in the evening. You might be just starting to suspect you have the condition. Or perhaps you are already into a lengthy battle against plantar fasciitis and you are not yet winning. Possibly, you have been trying to tough it out, carrying on with the usual activities and hoping it simply goes away. But it doesn't go away, and the pain persists.

To make matters worse, people close to you have no idea what you're going through. You've described your condition, but they don't seem to get it. How did you acquire it? Well, you're not really sure. It just seemed to come out of nowhere. You don't have a short sound bite to summarize its cause. Your explanation gets long, and they tune out. Maybe they think you sound like a hypochondriac. But the stabbing pain in the morning is real, the limping is real, the return of the soreness in the evening is real. And also real is the fact that you can no longer run or walk like you did, or stand on your two feet for any length of time. Until someone experiences plantar fasciitis, they can't understand the intricacies of your suffering.

If you're hobbled by plantar fasciitis, you naturally want to heal. But how long is the recovery time needed to recuperate from a bout of plantar fasciitis? There is no definite time frame. Your activity level, type of work you do, weight, footwear, age, flexibility, rest periods - or lack of them - between past exercise sessions, and the anatomy of your specific feet can all determine the recuperation time. As can the length of time you've had plantar fasciitis before you started to address it. Some folks recover in a couple of months, some take a year or more.

This brings up an important point. Advice on the subject can vary, but one expert source after another repeats a consistent theme: plantar fasciitis rarely goes away on its own. If you try to ignore it, and keep doing what you did to bring it on in the first place, plantar fasciitis will only get worse. You could develop other maladies as well, such as knee, hip or back conditions, as you change your normal gait to favor the injury. You must face the problem and take action to alleviate it. Initially ignoring the early symptoms was nearly a catastrophe for me. It added months to my recovery time. I wish I had started the recuperation steps and preventive measures sooner. Instead, I plowed ahead and tried to forget about it, hoping it would just disappear. It didn't. I had an early second chance to recover and I trampled over it. Don't make the same mistake.

Did I mention the silver lining in all of this? The time you spend repairing your ailing feet may bring about some unexpected side benefits. I definitely found this to be true during my plantar fasciitis ordeal.

To maintain some semblance of fitness and prevent weight gain, I turned to alternative exercises in place of running. I unearthed my bicycle, cleaned the cobwebs off, and started to use it again. As soon as

I could, I walked more regularly to burn calories. I gradually worked into a humble swimming routine, the first time I had used swimming for exercise in decades. Strength training was easier to work into my routine, and the results seemed to come easier when I wasn't logging so many miles training for the next running race. And last but not least, I buckled down and stretched on a regular basis. My muscles weren't as flexible as I thought they were. Once the stretching routine took effect, daily activities and workouts became easier. And it simply felt good to stretch.

The well-rounded fitness approach I turned to worked muscles in different ways and with an emphasis different from which they had become accustomed. It made me more flexible and gave my system a chance to recover. If you are already an avid runner, hiker, or walker, you may find the switch to a new regimen a welcome change. It may boost your strength and endurance in surprising ways. If you are new to exercise, this may be the jump start you need to venture down a more fit and solid path. In either case, your feet will thank you for it.

Want more good news? The recuperation plan found here will bring immediate improvement to the suffering caused by plantar fasciitis. Will it cure a person of it instantly? That's doubtful. If an instant fix for plantar fasciitis exists, it's not yet been discovered. But you will have less pain, better flexibility, more strength, and a lower chance of re-injury once you start on the steps detailed here. The positive effects will be realized right away. The healing will start right away. Thousands of past sufferers have proven this to be true. Hey, even I was a guinea pig for the cause. I field tested everything contained here, and it saved my feet.

Introduction

The hard-hitting, debilitating foot condition known as plantar fasciitis (pronounced "PLAN-ter fash-ee-I-tis") afflicts millions of people each year. According to the American Academy of Family Physicians, more than 600,000 outpatient visits result from plantar fasciitis annually, and that's in the United States alone. Plantar fasciitis plagues up to 10 percent of the entire population. Of all the foot problems people can acquire, plantar fasciitis is the most common, and is considered one of the most difficult from which to recover.

The hobbling symptoms of plantar fasciitis can affect workdays, shelve exercise routines, and sideline athletic endeavors. Functions normally taken for granted like walking and standing in place can become excruciating. Plantar fasciitis can cause regular life schedules to be thrown off and getting out of bed in the morning to become agony. Those that suffer from plantar fasciitis can experience the painful condition for weeks, months, or in some cases, years.

But despite the misery plantar fasciitis inflicts, it is often a preventable and highly treatable condition.

How exactly does plantar fasciitis manifest itself?

To begin with, your foot contains a thick, sturdy band of connective tissue which runs from your heel to the base of your toes. This tissue, called the plantar fascia, supports your foot's arch. It also surrounds and protects the related muscles and bones of your foot (see Figure 1). The level of toughness the plantar fascia exhibits is nothing short of incredible.

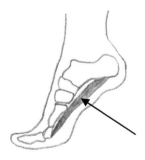

Figure 1: The plantar fascia (darkened area indicated by the arrow)

From the time you could walk, the plantar fascia has weathered the pounding of every step, every run, and every jump. It has rebounded when you've rushed down stairs, climbed steep inclines, and mowed the lawn. The plantar fascia has held its own when you've stood for hours. It has survived pickup basketball games, exercise sessions, and jogs around the lake. It has maintained its integrity when you've squeezed your feet into attractive but less-than-sensible shoes, then hurried across unyielding concrete sidewalks and floors at the mall. And it has done this for years and years. The average person takes 5,000 to 12,000 steps daily. Many of these steps are on hard, unforgiving surfaces, and each step puts a force on the feet that is about one and a half times that person's body weight. When running, your feet withstand more than three times this force. From childhood to adulthood, the plantar fascia has endured all this, held its own, and helped you stand, walk, and run.

Yet despite its durability, the plantar fascia has a marked weakness. It lacks flexibility. The plantar fascia is made of collagen, and collagen is not very elastic. So even though the plantar fascia is pretty rugged, when it is subjected to impact, stresses, and strains, it does not stretch to any great extent and then bounce back. Instead, the force it weathers from this repetitive trauma causes tiny tears to form along its surface. These micro-tears will eventually heal, if allowed to do so. But if the abuse continues without rest or remedy, your feet have no chance to recover from the existing tears. With unrelenting trauma, bad things can happen. The micro-tears can increase. The collagen of which the plantar fascia is composed degenerates. Inflammation of the plantar fascia follows and remains. The inflammation causes debilitating pain.

And plantar fasciitis has set in.

For the painful malady that plantar fasciitis becomes, it gives surprisingly little forewarning. Instead, it typically creeps up on its victim. Activities that have been done painlessly for years may become suddenly hindered, then impossible, with the onset of plantar fasciitis. The micro-tears were occurring, accumulating, and setting you up for a load of misery. Yet until the injury is firmly in place, it does not hint at its approach. Plantar fasciitis is particularly crafty in that way. And because of its insidious nature, it's sometimes hard for a person suffering from plantar fasciitis to determine what exactly caused it.

How can you tell if you have it? Plantar fasciitis causes pain on the underside of the foot, mostly in the heel, particularly at the heel's inside edge. The back of the heel may become quite tender as well. A slight swelling may occur where your heel meets your instep. Usually, most of the pain from plantar fasciitis occurs near the heel, since that is the spot where the plantar fascia is thinnest and where it withstands the most pressure. The first few steps taken after getting out of bed are generally the most painful. With these first steps of the day, you may feel a piercing sensation along with a pulling at your heel. The pain can be quite sharp, as if you just stepped on broken glass. As you move on with your day, the heel pain may lessen and often disappears. The discomfort can return, however, after prolonged walking and standing, and resting may only bring temporary relief. The pain can actually be more intense after resting. And even if all soreness disappears during the day, the tenderness may resume once again in the evening, even if you manage to stay off your feet.

You may also develop "heel spurs" as a result of the plantar fasciitis. Heel spurs are calcium deposits which result from the inflamed plantar fascia being pulled and strained where it attaches to the heel. The heel spurs form at the front of the heel and can be felt through palpitation. Heel spurs themselves do not hurt, and do not cause plantar fasciitis. They are instead a symptom of it.

So what did you do that was so wrong, that thrust such "abuse" on your feet? Did you force your feet to endure torture beyond anything they were designed to withstand? Possibly. But perhaps your actions were constructive; you became dedicated and got serious about exercise. There's a chance you maintained a positive, healthy workout regimen, where you got your heart rate up, worked your muscles, and burned calories. Maybe you were exercising to lose weight. Or, you may have simply performed your job, one which requires you to be on your feet for long periods of time. In short, plantar fasciitis affects very active people and completely sedentary people, and those with activity levels anywhere in between. Its victims come in all shapes and sizes, and in just about any age range. However, the following factors increase your risk of experiencing plantar fasciitis:

- **Extensive use of the feet.** This includes just about every activity you do on your feet, if done for very long periods of time or with great intensity. Working all day on your feet and running are common causes.

- **Excess weight.** Carrying just 15 or 20 pounds of extra weight greatly increases the odds of plantar fasciitis occurring.
- **A heavy body.** Unfortunately, the effects of impact and stress on the feet are still amplified by a fit but larger body. Muscle and bone do count; the laws of physics ensure that your feet can't tell the difference.
- **Hazardous shoes.** In other words, the choice of footwear usually based on fashion instead of comfort. Shoes with high heels, an extremely tight fit, a loose and floppy fit, very little cushioning, and those which don't support the foot's arch belong in this category.
- **Age.** A 20-year-old can acquire a case of plantar fasciitis, but a person's risk becomes greater after age 30 and especially once he or she reaches middle age.
- **Doing too much too soon** when embarking on an exercise routine.
- **Doing too much total exercise** without adequate rest. In other words, overtraining.
- **Flat feet.**
- **Highly-arched feet.**
- **Inflexible calf muscles and Achilles tendons.** Tightness in these areas is a huge contributor to plantar fasciitis, as it places extra strain on the plantar fascia.

Any of these factors sound familiar? If any describe you, your activities, or your footwear, rest assured you're not alone. Common characteristics and behaviors can cause the condition to rear its ugly head, so you may not have done anything that horrendous or atypical to acquire plantar fasciitis. That's one reason it's so widespread. The figure stated earlier, 600,000 people seeking help for plantar fasciitis each year, describes only outpatient visits. These are the folks who go to see a doctor for their foot condition. They're just the ones we know about. Those who choose home treatment, which is ultimately the way plantar fasciitis must be treated in most cases, do not figure into this number. The official estimate of 10 percent of the U.S. population affected by plantar fasciitis means about 30 million people at any given time are either current or former sufferers of the torturous foot condition.

Suffering from a widespread condition or not, make it your goal to become a *former* sufferer.

Luckily, some of the risk factors listed can be controlled and some behaviors changed to reduce the incidence of plantar fasciitis and to help your feet heal. As a matter of fact, as alluded to above, the majority of plantar fasciitis cases are resolved through conservative home treatment, as opposed to medical procedures like surgery.

I've mentioned this already but it bears repeating: the sooner you begin with corrective action, the quicker you will recuperate, the quicker you will realize healthy feet once again, and the sooner you'll be able to perform the activities you need to do and love to do without pain. Not to mention, the less damage you will incur on your injured feet by ignoring the condition.

I've included 30 action items to guide you through the healing process. Each action item is listed in its own short chapter, to ease navigation from item to item. I made extra efforts to state all descriptions with as little scientific jargon as possible. It would make no sense to wow you, the reader, with numerous technical terms and cumbersome medical terminology. You will not be overwhelmed with excessive information. This book is designed for you to pick up, flip through, get some good suggestions and a dose of encouragement, and get on with the business of fixing your feet.

All action items are non-medical, non-invasive home treatments. They're not risky, and they should not hurt. But following these remedial steps takes perseverance. Each person is unique, as is that person's daily routine, physical condition, foot structure, and past adventures and misadventures which have resulted in that person's present level of injury severity. Just a few of the action items may do the trick for you. Or you may need them all. My advice is to examine all 30. If you're under the care of a physician, by all means discuss these action items with him or her. If you're just getting started on your recovery from plantar fasciitis, prepare for a complex but rewarding journey. Recuperating from plantar fasciitis can be tricky; it's often a fine balancing act, with plenty of inaction as well as action, restraint as well as enthusiasm. But once you beat this thing, you'll appreciate your feet like never before.

Nobody knows how long your recovery period will last, but there is definitely one best time to start it: right now.

Had enough of your feet being injured? Then let's get going.

"The natural healing force within each one of us is the greatest force in getting well."

- Hippocrates

1

Make a Commitment

This first chapter includes no strengthening, stretching, or specific treatment advice of any kind. But it's just as important as more active physical measures. As a veteran of the plantar fasciitis ordeal, I must level with you: getting a case of plantar fasciitis to go away can pose a serious challenge. If you have already struggled with the condition for some time, I don't need to tell you this. If you have just started the plantar fasciitis healing process, embrace this idea early on, and dedicate yourself to your recovery.

You'll need every advantage you can get. After all, you cannot perform your healing process in a vacuum. You still need to walk. You may need to stand on your feet for long periods of time. You still get back on your feet after a night spent in bed, and still get in and out of a tub or shower. And each of these and numerous other actions can cause a slight reinjury to your feet; as the reinjuries accumulate, your feet can be prevented from healing in short order. So, you must consistently do many positive things while keeping the negative factors to a minimum. The more the odds can be tipped in your favor, the better.

Most people cannot stay off their feet indefinitely, and this probably includes you. And even if you could, the weakened state of your feet and legs as a result of this inactivity would end up making matters worse. You must keep moving and stay strong, yet stave off backward progress. Therein lies the complex puzzle which is recuperation from plantar fasciitis. The balance required to reduce the condition and heal from it makes for a delicate scenario.

You've acquired a condition that has no fix-it pill, no miracle cure, no definite recovery time line, and no single cause which can be blamed for its existence. And plantar fasciitis has a nasty habit of recurring once normal activities are resumed. It's going to take a serious commitment from you to bring your feet back to a normal, uninjured condition. And then keep them there.

I did not take plantar fasciitis seriously at first, and I pushed through the warning signs and tried to ignore them. It was as if I heard my car making strange noises, and just turned up the radio to drown out the sounds and wait for them to disappear. And I now believe that disregard added months to my recovery phase. Don't make the same mistake. Now is not the time to become complacent regarding your course of action for recovery.

Study the action items included in this book, and follow them consistently. As mentioned already, you may need just a few of the actions to make a full recovery, or you may need every single one. Each person is unique, so your recovery plan may be somewhat individualized. You might recover from your foot dilemma quickly, maybe in just a few weeks. But it may take you months, and maybe a year or more. Thousands of victims of plantar fasciitis have proven that lengthy recoveries are fairly common. And I'm willing to bet that a large percentage of these slow-to-heal sufferers delayed taking action to rectify their injuries, just as I did. Or just as risky, they jumped back into full, rigorous activity too soon.

This is hardly meant to be a statement of doom and gloom. Recovery happens. After I walked around timidly with intermittent shots of pain for months, getting back into running and completing a few races felt spectacular! No gold medalist ever felt better than I did when I crossed those finish lines. But to do it, I had to face reality, learn as much as I could about the condition, and immerse myself in the process needed for recovery. Admit to yourself the serious nature of the situation that has befallen you. Make the commitment to fix your feet. Stay on target, no matter how boring, futile, tiresome or strange the whole process may seem at first. Take action right away, be confident, be patient, be consistent, and your feet will heal much, much faster.

2

Back Off

The comedian Henny Youngman appeared on a TV program years ago, on stage firing off one liners left and right. Before he got to his well-known quips like, "I just flew into town, and boy are my arms tired," and "take my wife...please" he was fending off complaints from band members up on stage with him. As part of the skit, one fellow rotated his arm a little while wincing, and whined "Henny, it hurts when I go like that."

To which Henny replied, "Don't go like that."

Simple, isn't it? For the speediest recovery from plantar fasciitis, you must stop doing the activity which you suspect caused it in the first place, or at least reduce that activity as much as possible. It most likely won't be easy. If you love to hike or take long walks, ceasing these activities can be difficult to endure. If you are a dedicated runner, ceasing a running program can be grueling. You may feel pent up, cooped up, restless, and unfulfilled. To hang up your exercise ritual, even for a short time, may be unthinkable.

If you work on your feet, you face an even more complex scenario. In some ways, your feet are your fortune, and when adjusting a schedule and job duties with a boss and team members you may or may not experience a smooth transition.

But you must reduce the wear and tear on your feet, and that may mean making some tough choices and significant changes to a routine, at least temporarily. If you do not, you'll most likely hinder progress toward your recovery. Grind away on your feet as in the past, continue stubbornly ahead even when it hurts, and wear the same hazardous footwear that you've been wearing, and the plantar fasciitis condition may in fact never heal.

This advice is hard to take, I know. But this is where commitment comes in. Remember commitment? Sometimes it entails gung ho enthusiasm for new strengthening exercises and stretches, active rehab, things you can do with vigor. But sometimes it means denial. Sometimes it means backing off. Sometimes it's boring. It's difficult to resist the temptation to jump back in too soon. But to speed healing and avoid reinjury, you have to surrender to the need for rest. If you do all other parts of the recovery plan faithfully but continue stressing your injury, you are in a sense shooting yourself in the foot. (Sorry, bad analogy.)

In all seriousness, come to terms with the fact that your plantar fasciitis condition requires some significant rest, and avoidance of those factors which caused it in the first place, however inconvenient this is to you. Avoid subjecting yourself to further aggravation. Give your feet a break and give them a chance to heal. The effectiveness of the upcoming actions will increase several times over if you do.

3

Wear Protective Shoes

You will need to plant your feet in a supportive, durable, resilient pair of shoes as soon as possible to minimize further damage to your plantar fascia. Once you've got the shoe piece of the puzzle figured out, you'll have made great strides in activating the healing process. Good shoes can protect your feet like a dream, and bad ones can sabotage them like a nightmare. In fact, dangerous shoes may have landed you on the plantar fasciitis roster in the first place.

Although a sales rep at a reputable shoe store can help you work out the details, here are a few things to look for as you seek new footwear:

- **Flexibility.** Make sure the shoe bends in the front half, where the ball of the foot will be when the shoe is worn. It should not bend in the middle or way back closer to the heel. In other words, your shoe should not bend in any area where your foot does not normally bend. If it does, that shoe's support will be marginal. Conversely, if the shoe barely bends at all, rule it out, as an overly-stiff shoe will be detrimental to your feet.
- **Stiff Heel Counter.** The back of the shoe where it engulfs your heel should fit firm and snug. Make sure your heel doesn't slide up and down.
- **Proper Fit for Your Feet...Right Now.** Have your feet measured before purchasing your next pair of shoes. Like most parts of our bodies, the feet change with age and the rigors of time. The current shoe size you need may be different than what you wore in the past. The width of your feet should be measured in addition to their length.
- **Arch Support.** Sufficient backbone where the shoe supports your arch is critical. Ensure that the shoe is not flimsy in this area and does not flatten out as you walk.
- **Low Heel.** This one is obvious. No more high heels or dashing boots that jack the back of your foot way up. Lose the pointy toes also.

- **A Little Room to Move.** You'll want a small amount of space in your shoes, both in terms of length and width, so your feet will be comfortable and blood can flow easily. Make sure your new shoes are not too roomy but not too tight either. This is especially important as the day progresses, since your feet will swell slightly as time goes on. For this very reason, the best time to try on a pair of shoes is later in the day.
- **A Design to Match High-Arched or Low-Arched Feet.** If you have a high arch, your foot type is somewhat stiff and requires more cushioning. If you have a low arch, your foot type will benefit from a more rigid shoe with "motion control" design.
- **A Good Fit and Feel Immediately.** A pair of shoes that aligns correctly with your feet should feel comfortable upon trying them on. Don't assume that the shoes will break in and accommodate your feet with time. They probably won't.

Oh, and make sure to replace your worn out shoes. Yes, even your favorite ones. Favorite old shoes, even those with no support left in them, can be set aside for a while and then somehow find their way back onto injured, recuperating feet. Acquiring new, solid-performing shoes is half of the footwear equation. Banish the old faithful but beat up shoes; they can put your feet back in danger. Throw them away if they appear to be mostly degraded. If they seem to be in usable condition but not intact enough for serious exercise, you can give them away to charity and still feel good about parting ways with them. And they may in fact work for someone else just fine. It could be that those shoes are just not right for your feet and circumstances.

For runners, some experts recommend replacing shoes every 500 miles. Other experts say replace them every 300 or 400 miles. For walkers, add about 100 miles to these figures at most. The owner of an old and loyal pair can generally tell if support from those shoes is waning. If you have a pair of shoes that have served you well, but fit the description of "waning support," make your peace, bid them farewell, and get yourself some new ones.

4

Avoid Going Barefoot

Like a fighter of yesteryear's hands exposed to the brutality of a bare-knuckle bout, traipsing around barefoot with a case of plantar fasciitis will pummel your injured feet. Protecting the existing injury is as important as the rehab activities you'll soon do. One way to provide protection is to keep them safely nestled in a pair of supportive shoes, even when you're at home. The plantar fascia already will bear the brunt of walking and standing activities, and maneuvering around while barefoot will increase this strain.

A pair of slippers or socks will not be adequate here. Use walking or running shoes, as they will support your arch and protect your heel. Upon stepping out of bed in the morning, step right into the shoes. After a shower, do the same thing. It may seem annoying or feel funny at first, but it doesn't take long to get in the habit.

You may want to get a new pair of shoes for the express purpose of wearing them indoors. The shoes won't get worn down from usage outside the home and will therefore remain in pristine condition with optimum support.

One caveat to this advice: plan on wearing shoes at all times in the home just for the short-term. I wore running shoes indoors myself for several months, and it definitely helped. My feet were shielded from extra wear and tear, and they had a better chance to heal. But I noticed one big difference after this length of time: my feet seemed noticeably weaker. Some of the muscles had simply atrophied. I had been doing plenty of walking, so inactivity was not to blame. The motion, flexion, and adjustments of a human foot are activated differently when barefoot than when in shoes; a barefoot walking motion keeps feet strong in a way that moving about in shoes simply cannot. Humankind has moved in bare feet to some extent for thousands of years. Going barefoot has its place. It's just not ideal while your plantar fasciitis condition is in its acute phase.

When you feel sharp pain in your feet, keep them protected in a good pair of shoes, even while at home. After your recuperation moves along and the pain is subsiding, slowly wean yourself off the shoes, and move around barefoot from time to time.

5

Use Cushioning on the Shower Floor

This discovery was bred out of necessity, and I felt it was a small but valuable piece of advice to share. I had read several times from experts the good advice of stepping straight into a pair of supportive shoes when getting out of bed. I also listened to the advice to keep wearing the shoes indoors, and put on another good pair for walking outside. Basically, I heard the message loud and clear to keep those aching feet protected at all times with durable shoes. And it worked, for the most part.

But what about in the shower? A hard bathtub floor or shower floor can be a brutal surface when your feet are in pain. By the end of some showers I'd be wincing once again from the grind of my heels on the unyielding floor material.

More than once I came across the advice "Don't go barefoot - not even in the shower." Wait a minute. I want to do whatever is best for my aching feet, but...wear my running shoes in the shower? Hmm. I opted for a different method.

After trying a couple of ideas, I found one convenient solution to this chink in the armor. I used a flat foam pad, the type sold for just a few dollars for sitting in stadiums, parks, at outdoor concerts, in the woods when hunting, etc. It's sometimes called a thermal seat. It provided all the cushioning necessary, was lightweight, and it dried easily.

Naturally, any other piece of material with similar cushioning would work fine. Even a boat cushion would fit the bill. This may sound strange, but who can argue with an extra pain barrier?

Could you get by without a foam pad on the shower or bathtub floor? Yes, you could. But why leave any stone unturned? For the same reason nobody sleeps on a bed made out of concrete, it makes sense to provide your feet with a cushioned layer when standing on a solid tub floor. You'll save a little wear and tear on your injury, and your feet will feel better after a shower or bath. The foam pads are inexpensive and multi-purpose. They are sold in department stores and online by various sporting goods dealers. Get one and give it a try.

6

Wear a Night Splint

One of the absolute best steps you can take to recover from plantar fasciitis is to acquire and wear a night splint. Commercial night splints are padded, generally comfortable devices you wear while you sleep. They are simple and painless to use. The night splint resembles a big boot with an open front. You just step into the splint and tether it to your foot for the night with a few Velcro straps. Then, you can pretty much forget about it until the next morning. It's unlikely that a night splint will disturb your sleep.

A night splint is effective because it keeps the foot in a relatively straight position and at a 90-degree angle with the leg. Normally the foot assumes a somewhat slack, curving position while sleeping. A kind of "fetal position" if you will. This action is natural and usually harmless. But with a foot recuperating from plantar fasciitis, scar tissue begins to form overnight. And it takes place while the foot is in the described relaxed position. Once the foot "uncurls" and straightens and you take your first steps of the day, the new scar tissue tears; the plantar fascia gets strained, and the micro-tears recur. This tearing causes the majority of pain most plantar fasciitis sufferers feel with those early morning steps. A night splint largely eliminates this chain of events, as it keeps your foot somewhat straightened as you sleep and the plantar fascia stretched (the scar tissue formed will therefore not be torn when you get out of bed, since the foot is already in the flexed position).

In addition, a night splint helps keep your calf muscles slightly stretched through the night. Discussed at length later in this book, flexible calf muscles are an integral part of your recuperation from plantar fasciitis.

You can purchase a night splint from a large number of physical therapy equipment and medical device dealers, either from a retail outlet or online. Night splints generally run from $70.00 to $110.00 or so. For further advice and explanation of different models, you would want to visit a walk-in location. I ordered mine online, and it worked out quite well. I only wish I had ordered a couple of them, since I suffered from plantar fasciitis in both feet. I wore my night splint on my left foot primarily, as it seemed the more injured of the two. In hindsight, it now seems like a comedy of errors, as I began switching the splint from one foot to the next on alternating nights.

If you're serious about overcoming plantar fasciitis, get a night splint and wear it. If you suffer from the condition in both feet, break down and buy two. You'll be surprised how much a night splint aids in your healing, and getting up in the morning will be much less of a pain.

7

Ice the Injured Area

The plantar fasciitis condition is an injury, and like most injuries, swelling can occur in the immediate area. This inflammation will not only increase discomfort, it will limit normal motion and impede the healing process. The most immediate and effective method to reduce the inflammation is to apply ice to the injury. Ice will enhance your healing and deaden some of the pain. It will help remove detrimental fluids and allow nutrients to enrich the injured site. This will encourage the repair process and help your feet heal sooner.

Various methods are available to deliver ice applications to the injury, such as commercial ice packs, a plastic bottle filled with water and allowed to freeze, or ice cubes wrapped in a towel. Another good and very convenient method is simply a bag of frozen vegetables. Frozen corn kernels and peas are both ideal, as their rounded shape makes for a comfortable texture when you do the icing. The individual pieces in the bag move freely and will mold to the shape of your foot. And they can be used over and over. The procedure can be as easy as placing the frozen veggies on the floor, then resting your feet on them as you sit in a comfortable chair. Unless it causes pain, you can work a gentle ice massage into the treatment by moving your feet against the ice pack, slowly and gently.

Do not apply ice or frozen items directly against your skin. This can cause ice burns and damage to your skin. Place a moist towel between your skin and the cold pack to avoid any such danger.

Do not overdo it with icing. Ice treatment of the tender area for 10 minutes at a given time is usually plenty. You can actually damage the tissue if you ice it excessively. Do the icing twice a day in the early stage of plantar fasciitis, or if a reinjury of your feet ever crops up. Once you're well on your way to healing, once a day should be enough.

Icing will be especially valuable if you have just been on your feet for a long time, or right after walking or running. Do it immediately following these activities for best results.

Speaking of walking, running, and reinjury: if you do at some point jump back into activity with a little too much vigor and suffer a reinjury, make sure to apply ice to the area as soon as you can. The benefit of icing an acute injury diminishes after 48 hours or so. Catch the recurrence in time with ice treatment, and the damage will be greatly minimized.

So keep icing in mind for a convenient, low cost, and effective form of therapy. Sit back, relax, and let your feet chill out.

A Word About Stretching

No absolute verdict has ever been reached on the very best method with which to stretch muscles of the human body. If a person researched the topic until locating 100 articles or books on stretching, I think that person would find some glaring discrepancies. Probably 30 or 50 or 70 different takes on the number of repetitions, length of time to hold a stretch, stretching a cold muscle vs. a warmed-up muscle, and how far to stretch an inflexible muscle would appear. Overwhelming agreement amongst the experts on stretching does not seem to exist.

I don't have the final answer on stretching, but I know a couple of things:

Stretching can help you recover from plantar fasciitis, and
Stretching can injure you.

Over the years, I got into the bad habit of never stretching. My best guess is that this lack of stretching helped me acquire plantar fasciitis in the first place. But once I started stretching on a regular basis, the healing process accelerated. I mean, really accelerated. The healing seemed to take place several times faster. And on walks and hikes where the soreness would recur, taking the time to stretch again would usually reduce the pain or make it go away completely. Stretching is a good thing, and most experts on the subject agree that it is not only helpful but imperative to stretch to resolve a case of plantar fasciitis.

But if you stretch a muscle with too much force and in too much of a hurry, the muscle can tear. And your injury problem will then become compounded. So keep three words in mind for a successful stretching venture: *Consistent. Patient. Gentle.*

Stretch regularly, at least once a day, as you help yourself heal from plantar fasciitis. A few times a week will not be enough. And try not to hurry. You must hold a stretch for it to work, and you might find yourself becoming a bit bored. Practice patience. And above all, be gentle when stretching. If it hurts, back off. If a stretch goes no further without discomfort, don't force the stretch past that point. Ever. Be gentle and you won't injure yourself while stretching.

How long should you hold a stretch? Over the years I've heard figures from two seconds all the way up to sixty seconds, and a wide variety within that range. Basically, they've all worked for me. As long as I did the stretches in the first place, and didn't get too rough while doing them. I've listed the very general estimate in this book of holding a stretch 15-20 seconds, then repeating that stretch three or four times. Why? It's worked for me. If you find holding a stretch shorter or longer than 15-20 seconds works better, then do it that way. Experiment and find the best duration of stretching for you personally. Just remember to be consistent, patient, and gentle, and your stretching endeavor will be effective.

8

Stretch Your Calf Muscles

Flexibility in your calf muscles is so crucial to reducing the injured condition of your feet that its importance cannot be overstated. Limberness in this area is vital to recovery from plantar fasciitis. The following analogy may help in understanding this.

Think of the underside of the foot as a bow; the arch is the bow limbs and the plantar fascia is the string. Tight calf muscles pull on the heel cord, and make the "bow limbs" attempt to straighten. Straighten more than they were designed to, in fact. This exerts quite a strain on the "string," or in real life, on the plantar fascia (see Figure 2). While under this increased tension, the introduction of any of the other factors which contribute to plantar fasciitis (bad shoes, excessive exercise, excessive weight, lack of rest, etc.) the damage becomes exacerbated. Already embattled with the other risk factors, the plantar fascia undergoes extra strain and impact from tightness in the calf. Tight calf muscles interfere with normal foot mechanics, and your plantar fascia suffers as a consequence.

The combination of inflexible calves with other risk factors can often lead to a full-blown case of plantar fasciitis. In contrast, the introduction of flexibility in the calves removes a big liability for getting the condition in the first place. If you already suffer from it, plantar fasciitis is less likely to stick around once your calf area becomes flexible. Make your calves more limber and reduce the strain on your plantar fascia.

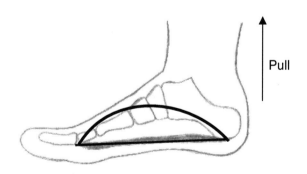

Pull

Figure 2: Illustration of pull on the plantar fascia

Remember, think gentle. While stretching your calf, you're also stretching the very region that is injured, so take care to not worsen the condition by stretching too vigorously. That said, you may find yourself amazed at the reduction in tenderness and the return of durability your feet experience once flexibility in the calf area sets in. Dedicate yourself to this simple stretching routine and realize big dividends.

Two primary stretches can be used to increase flexibility in the calf area.

Seated Calf Stretch

While sitting on a comfortable surface, extend both legs in front of you. Reach forward carefully and grab your toes and the balls of your feet. (You can bend your knees as necessary; the stretch still works with bent knees.) Ever so mildly, pull the top of your foot back toward you, to the point that you feel a stretch begin (see Figure 3). You should feel the effect in your calf and in the Achilles tendon at the back of the heel (you'll also feel a stretch in your hamstrings if you're keeping your legs somewhat straight). Pull no further; hold that position and let the stretch take place. Maintain the stretch for 15-20 seconds, and repeat the process three or four times.

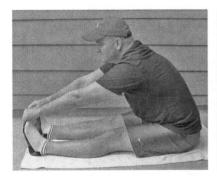 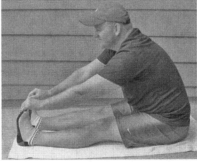

Figure 3: Seated calf stretch starting position (left picture) and stretched position (right picture)

If you presently have some difficulty reaching your feet in this position, as many people do, first wrap a towel around the bottom of your feet, then extend your legs in front of you. With this extra reach in place, proceed with the calf stretch in the same way as described above. Position the towel around the balls of your feet, and initiate the stretch with a light touch (see Figure 4). Once you feel the stretch take effect, stretch no further and hold it at that point. Maintain the stretch for 15-20 seconds, and repeat the process three or four times.

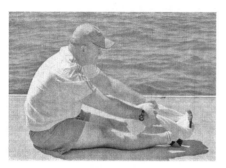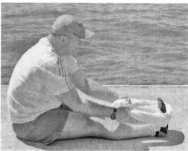

Figure 4: Seated calf stretch using a towel; starting position (left picture) and stretched position (right picture)

Lunge Position Stretch

This stretch shines due to both its effectiveness and its versatility. You won't need to don special exercise clothes or lie down on the floor. It can be done just about anywhere and at almost any time, regardless of what you're wearing. Furthermore, items like a dresser, a chair, or even a tree or a wall can be used to brace yourself as you conduct the stretch. The ready availability of the lunge position stretch makes it ideal to do while out on a walk, at work, or before and after any exercise session.

Place your hands on one of the stabilizing objects described above and the leg to be stretched set back behind you, foot flat on the floor. The front leg will be slightly bent at the knee. To execute the stretch, let your forward leg flex a bit more at the knee, and maneuver your hips slightly forward. Gently move into the stretch (see Figure 5). Once you feel the stretch in the calf area and the Achilles tendon (at the back of the heel) go no further and hold the stretch. Hold for 15-20 seconds. Repeat the sequence three or four times.

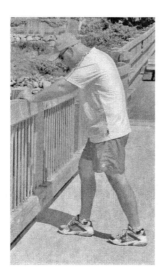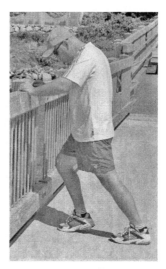

Figure 5: Lunge position stretch starting position (left picture) and stretched position (right picture)

9

Stretch Your Arches

In addition to stretching out your calf area to reduce strain on the plantar fascia, you can stretch the arch itself. This will make the plantar fascia slightly more flexible, reducing the pulling and strain experienced where it attaches at the heel. The result will be reduced tenderness and less swelling in the heel and arch.

The procedure for the arch stretch is as follows: while sitting, set the foot across your opposite knee. Grab your toes and the ball of your foot, and gently bend the foot back (see Figure 6). If you are in the early throes of the plantar fasciitis ordeal, don't expect to bend your foot back very far before you feel some soreness. Stop the stretch if you feel pain at any point. Ease up, and stretch your arch to a lesser degree. If you attempt to stretch the arch further than it's ready to, you could injure yourself further. Developing flexibility anywhere in the body is a gradual process, and nowhere is this truer than in the arch. Hold the stretch for about 15-20 seconds, and repeat the process three or four times.

I recommend doing this stretch a little later in the morning, vs. first thing upon awakening. All parts of your body will be stiffened from sleep, especially your arch. After doing some early morning stretching (detailed later), you may want to move around for awhile and then do the arch stretch. Your feet will then be warmed up from stepping and walking, and may be more receptive to being stretched. If you do decide to stretch your arches early in the morning, before walking, do so with extra care.

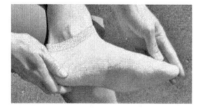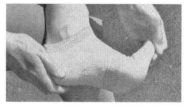

Figure 6: Arch stretch starting position (left picture) and stretched position (right picture)

10

Stretch Your Hamstrings

Tight hamstrings can be tough to live with. Not only do inflexible hamstrings put these long, strong muscles in the back of your thigh themselves at risk, but they also cause undue tension on other body parts. The most publicized by-product of stiff hamstrings is the extra wear and tear they cause on the lower back. Similarly, tight hamstrings place extra stress on the plantar fascia.

It's a somewhat complex series of events. Lack of hamstring flexibility can cause less-than-ideal leg motions. One example is over-flexion of the knee. When the knee over-flexes, the effect travels down the leg, and results in excess flexion of the ankle as well. This causes extra stress on the Achilles tendon, which then exerts extra pull on the heel bone and plantar fascia.

Simply put, like tight calf muscles and Achilles tendons, inflexible hamstrings are quite taxing on the plantar fascia. Allowing them to stay inflexible means the progress in your recovery can be hindered. Regular stretching can remedy this situation.

A number of good hamstring stretches are out there, and here's one which is effective, safe, and somewhat relaxing.

While on your back, raise one leg, keeping it bent at the knee just a bit, hold the leg behind the knee, and slowly, gently extend your leg (see Figure 7). This will stretch the hamstring area. Expect the hamstring to be a little tight if you have not stretched it regularly.

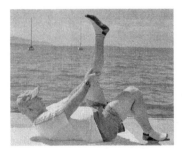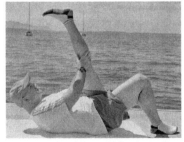

Figure 7: Supine hamstring stretch starting position (left picture) and stretched position (right picture)

A slight variation to this procedure is to wrap a towel around the center of your foot, vs. holding your leg with your hands. Pull carefully on the towel as you extend your leg, stopping and holding the position once you feel a stretch begin (see Figure 8).

Hold the stretch for about 15-20 seconds, and repeat the process three or four times. Remember to go easy when stretching any of your muscles, the hamstrings included. Be patient as well, as it may take a few sessions to see noticeable changes in your range of motion. Repeat this procedure once every day at least. Twice is better.

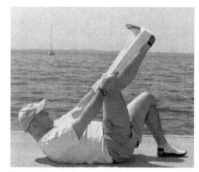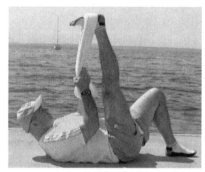

Figure 8: Supine hamstring stretch using a towel; starting position (left picture) and stretched position (right picture)

Of all the endeavors listed in this book, developing hamstring flexibility is one of the most beneficial to your entire body. It assists in ease of movement in just about every motion your body can perform. And it feels good, almost a relief, when tight hamstrings get good and loosened up. In addition, supple and flexible hamstrings are better protected and are less likely to become "pulled" when you're active. So make a commitment to regularly stretch this area, and enjoy the smoother, more efficient functioning realized by improving this key muscle group.

11

Stretch First Thing in the Morning

It's no secret that the time immediately following a full night's sleep will be when your body experiences the most stiffness of the entire day. That stiffness includes the plantar fascia, which tends to tighten overnight. That makes early morning the most necessary time of the day to perform some key stretches before moving about. Stretching now will eliminate some of that stiffness and make you more limber. This in turn will help keep your feet safe as you seize the day.

However, early morning is also the time of day where safe stretching is the trickiest.

If you're like me, it's enough just to get up to your feet from the bed without joints all over your body popping and cracking. You've been in bed all night, and you're going to be a little tight. A full flexibility routine before you even stand up from the bed is not only difficult, it can be dangerous. Stretching can be an invaluable part of a plantar fasciitis recovery regimen, but you don't want to injure yourself with the same stretches you now count on to ease your pain.

I highly recommend sticking to just two early morning stretches. The first stretch: while on your back, raise one leg, keeping it bent at the knee just a bit, hold the leg behind the knee, and slowly, gently perform the supine hamstring stretch, covered in the previous chapter. You almost certainly will be tighter, much more so, than when you do this stretch in the middle of the day or in the evening, so keep that in mind. Hold it for a while, about 15-20 seconds, and then slowly straighten your knee a bit more. Feel the stretch effect in your hamstring area. Repeat it three or four times, then add some ankle flexion to the stretch. Bring your toes very slowly toward your shin. This stretches your calf and Achilles tendon. Again, hold it for a while, and then relax it. Repeat this three or four times. Then switch legs, and use the same process to prepare your other leg for the day ahead.

The second stretch: get to your feet and lean on the side of the bed, or grab a dresser or chair if they are close by. (Step directly into your indoor shoes if your feet are in the acute phase of your plantar fasciitis challenge - the phase where you are advised to wear shoes at all times.) Proceed with the same motion as the lunge stretch, described earlier in Chapter 8. Perform three or four repetitions with this stretch also, using your bed, dresser, or chair to lean against. Of course, if the wall is right by your bed, just use that. The idea here is to avoid walking all over before the stretches are done. The less weight bearing movement you do at this point the better. Get your hamstrings, calf muscles, and Achilles loosened in a gingerly manner before you adventure about. The most damage can be done to your injured plantar fascia upon those first morning steps if the related mechanisms are still stiffened from sleep.

The early morning stretch will be of less importance if you wear a night splint as described in Chapter 6, but even so, a simple, careful stretch can still help for those first few steps. And please, recognize if there was ever a time for slow motion stretching, early morning is that time. Ease your body through the stretch sequence, and don't rush it. Be patient and go easy on yourself. With that said, stretching your legs as described can make getting into the swing of things much easier and less painful first thing in the morning. It's like an archer fitting the bow with a longer string, so the limbs can relax.

12

Bike for Exercise

You may find yourself in a quandary regarding exercise due to your plantar fasciitis ordeal. Perhaps you were in the good habit of walking for exercise, and that routine has now been tripped up by your foot injury. You struggle to walk around the kitchen, much less around the park. Even walking on a treadmill might hurt, despite its built-in cushion. Or if you like to hike, the reality of foot and heel tenderness is even more evident, given the steep nature and unpredictable texture of many trails.

And if you are in the acute stage of plantar fasciitis, subjected to frequent stabs of pain nipping at your heels, let's not even mention running. The pounding down of your bodyweight, coupled with the sheer number of footfalls realized on an average run, translates into a taxing experience for your feet. Yet you still want to keep moving, stay strong, and burn some calories. You may return to walking, hiking, and yes, even running in due time. But for now you need an alternative exercise source. What to do?

Consider biking.

Biking is a great cardiovascular workout. It is a non-weight bearing exercise, so stress and jarring on your feet will be minimal. In addition, biking will provide incredible quadriceps conditioning. Your hamstrings, buttocks, hips, and calves will get in on the action too. It will help you improve endurance and strength, and add to the muscle mass in your legs and lower body. And with any gain in solid body mass, you will burn more energy, even while resting. This quiet sizzle of calories will help you avoid an increase in body fat; it may even help you lose some. And any weight you can shed will mean that much less force on your feet, helping to speed your recovery and prevent the condition's recurrence.

You can ride a bike with intensity, simulating a competitor on the Tour de France, but for moderate aerobic and strength training, feel free to ride casually. You'll still get plenty of exercise. As a matter of fact, once you slow way down, the resistance experienced to get back up to speed will be greater than if you were going fast, since you've lost forward momentum. The aerobic training and strength development will be substantial, and so will the energy you burn for weight control.

A couple of points in terms of technique when biking, to protect your body. Make sure your knees go pretty much straight up and down; don't angle them outwards, away from the bike. The straight up and down motion will exert less strain on your feet as well as your knees. Also, push the pedals with the middle of the foot vs. the ball of the foot. The mechanics of pushing with the ball of the foot will stress the plantar fascia. Pumping the pedals with the midfoot, on the other hand, will exert little strain here.

Any benefits realized by riding a bike outdoors can also be attained by working out on an exercise bike. In most ways, your body won't know the difference. Jump on either type of bike and move those pedals. You'll build endurance and some key leg muscles while you fry up lots of calories at the same time.

13

Walk for Exercise

To keep moving, relieve stress, burn calories, and hasten your foot recovery, do some walking. You should of course go easy if your plantar fasciitis condition is in the acute stage. But make sure you go. Walking is a readily available, versatile, convenient, and inexpensive activity. It gives some folks peace of mind and as a result helps them improve their mood, stay positive, and even sleep better. And for such a seemingly gentle endeavor, it's quite effective in delivering results in terms of a workout.

If you are a runner, this chapter could be titled "Walk Instead of Run for Exercise." While in plantar fasciitis recovery mode, you may want to avoid the high impact of running, and walk instead. Or at least consider replacing running with walking in the most acute phase of your injury. If you are not very active, but possibly acquired plantar fasciitis by standing on your feet for long periods of time, this may be a call for you to get more active and invigorate the muscles of your lower legs, ankles, and feet. Walking can greatly assist in some serious conditioning and strengthening of those areas, while subjecting you to very little impact.

The lack of impact realized while walking can be a huge plus. While walking, the force exerted upon your feet is only about one and a half times your body weight. While running, by comparison, your feet often endure up to bodyweight times ten.

The payoff in terms of calorie burn and conditioning gained while walking fast are undeniable, but you don't have to speed walk or race walk. In fact, when you walk slowly, momentum doesn't continue to carry you forward as it does when you walk very fast, so your muscles work a bit more to lift you and propel you from a near dead stop. In truth, slow, medium, and brisk walking speeds will all provide a good workout. Walk at the speed with which you're most comfortable. The key is to get out and do it. And if you ever find yourself becoming out of breath, slow down. You just don't have to push yourself that hard to reap walking's benefits.

Despite the low level of impact, you'll still want to walk in good form and with a normal foot strike. (More on this in Chapter 24.) It can be tempting when suffering with ailing feet to limp or favor one side over the other. Resist making this mistake. Especially, be sure to avoid walking on the outside of the foot. This foot position may seem to give the injured areas of your feet a rest, but in fact creates significant strain on the plantar fascia, in particular at the point where it attaches to the heel bone. To make matters worse, other portions of your foot may then suffer injury, increasing your recovery dilemma.

Even though walking is relatively easy on your feet, increase the distance you walk gradually. You may feel gung ho about your walking program, ready to exceed past distances, explore new places, burn even more calories, and strengthen your feet. This type of enthusiasm is a great thing, but use common sense at the same time. Walking will not stress your feet like running, rugged hiking, or the fast stops and starts experienced in many sports. But it is still serious exercise. Walking will tax your muscles and connective tissue, which is actually one reason it's beneficial to you. But it can be overdone, especially when plantar fasciitis is in its early stages. So if a given distance results in increased pain, vs. simple muscle soreness, cut back on the length of your walk for the time being.

If you read or hear something to the effect that a person should walk at least six days a week for thirty or forty minutes at a time minimum, take the advice with a grain of salt. You may or may not be ready for that type of exertion. Be enthused but cautious. Use a gradual approach. You'll work up to greater frequency and distance with time. I've read the suggested amount of 10% by which to increase your distance per week, but that's just a ballpark figure. You can lengthen your walks by even less than that each week and still make good progress. Or, if you find a walk location or routine you really like, don't feel pressure to increase the distance at all. Regular and consistent walks are far more important than occasional long ones. That should be your priority for a walking program, not setting new records each week.

If you can only walk five or eight minutes at a time, due to time constraints or your level of injury, try to repeat these time increments a few times a day. The positive effects of walking can be realized in a cumulative sense. Five walking outings of five minutes each is roughly as beneficial as a contiguous twenty-five minute session. If short walks are all you can fit in to your day, take heart and keep at it.

Keep in mind this sinister characteristic of plantar fasciitis: pain tends to disappear as exercise progresses. This may give you a false sense of security, tempting you to subject your feet to exertion for which they are not ready. If your injury is in the acute stage, where pain is quite sharp first thing in the morning, you can inflict upon your vulnerable feet additional damage by trying too much too soon. Resist that urge. As it relates to the old adage "First we crawl, then we walk," make sure you don't walk yourself into needing to crawl. (Sound drum roll and cymbal.)

See Chapter 24, "Maintain Low Impact Form," to minimize any additional trauma your feet might experience as you make strides to get back in the game. Remember, plantar fasciitis recovery is a tricky business. You need to keep moving, but avoid doing too much at the same time. And just as importantly, make sure you walk in good, supportive shoes. Chapter 3 covers shoe selection in greater detail.

With that said, make a conscious effort to walk more, and plan the outings according to the amount your feet will allow. It will strengthen and tone your entire lower body, including those crucial muscles of the lower leg and foot. It may also help you sleep better, lift your spirits, and encourage you to stay committed to your overall recovery program. Include some variety, challenge yourself slowly but surely, and enjoy yourself.

14

Swim for Exercise

If you want an exercise that is easy on your feet, subjects you to no impact, strengthens your entire body, and burns calories like crazy, go swimming.

As mentioned earlier in this book, I turned to swimming for exercise after my feet became stricken with plantar fasciitis. And it was then and only then that I reintroduced myself to it. I took swimming lessons as a kid, and went swimming from time to time my entire life. But it was mostly for fun, in a pool jumping off a high dive a few times, or at a public beach, swimming out to the diving raft and back after doing a couple of cannonballs. So I certainly am no expert on swimming techniques or strokes. I cannot outline a swimming regimen for fitness, but I know from experience even a very short session will intensely work out a person's muscles and cardiovascular system.

Here was my experience when I introduced swimming into my fitness routine. Keep in mind I was a fairly serious, middle of the pack recreational runner leading up to my injury. In the preceding twelve months I had completed a half marathon and two ten-mile races. So a pretty decent fitness capacity was in place. I could no longer run due to my aching feet, but I got back on my mountain bike, as well as an exercise bike, with regularity. I could crank out about an hour of vigorous biking without any danger of collapsing. I continued to lift weights as I had for years, so I was maintaining my strength. I felt I was in pretty good shape. Until I started swimming.

Within five minutes of my first swim session, I was ready to fold like wilted lettuce. My limbs were exhausted and my lungs ached for air. I couldn't believe how much energy a few laps consumed. What a workout! With time, I added a minute or two to each swim, learned to slow down, and worked on proper form. And when I was too tired to actually swim any longer, I found I could grab the side of the pool and just flutter kick a while, adding another minute or two at the end of the workout.

If you have experience as a competitive swimmer or triathlete, you're probably laughing at this. But for a person who has not used it for exercise, the fitness demands of swimming are no joke. Even if you are in good condition for activities like biking, walking, and running, a swim can tax your aerobic and anaerobic abilities like nothing else. Swimming is an activity all its own. And for such a high value strengthening and calorie-consuming activity, swimming is surprisingly easy on the joints.

During my swim-for-exercise project, my feet experienced no ill effects from swimming. They actually got to rest a little, even though my system was going through grueling workouts. To sum it up, swimming = lots of exertion with zero impact.

My swimming and overall fitness improved, and I actually ended up using swimming as an integral part of aerobic training to later run a five-mile race. At the time, I could only run short distances safely, so I needed other options to build my endurance back up. I didn't want to bike for every workout, and thus found swimming to be the perfect answer for this needed training boost.

If you don't know how to swim, or it's been a long time since you have, consider swimming lessons. This period of recuperation on which you have embarked can be a time to try new things, and swimming might be a good challenge to tackle. And while you learn, you'll build endurance and strength while expending quite a few calories. Maybe it will turn into a life-long activity for you, who knows.

Closely related to swimming is *deep water running*, which simulates running on land while wearing a flotation device. I've not yet tried this, but many athletes and coaches swear by it as a method of cross-training and injury recovery. Consider looking into a deep water running class at a local university or community pool. It could serve you well as a workout and an alternative to swimming if you're looking to mix up your activities further. And like swimming, your feet will suffer no impact whatsoever.

For a total body workout that spares your feet of any abuse, dive into the swimming routine and get some serious exercise.

15

Strengthen Your Calf Muscles

To help stabilize the motion of your ankles and feet, work on building strength in your calf muscles. Strong muscles in your calf area assist in controlling the action of the foot's strike, roll, and push-off with each step. The stronger your calves are, the more your feet will be stabilized during this process.

Strengthening your calf muscles will deliver the extra benefit of greater endurance: you'll be able to work, exercise and stand in place longer without tiring your lower legs. Your feet in turn will receive better support and protection. This will make things like maintaining weight, getting through a workday on your feet, and having fun outdoors more attainable.

Your calves get worked during just about any movement you make on your feet or with your legs. Walking, biking, running, playing tennis, and climbing stairs are just a few examples of activities which involve your calf muscles, as well as many other muscles simultaneously. To isolate the calves and work just them primarily, you can use two simple yet effective exercises. They are as follows:

Standing Calf Raise

There's not a lot to describe here. For starters, while standing, you may want to hold on to a railing, table, or the back of a chair for balance. Then, raise yourself up so your heels leave the ground, and you balance on the balls of your feet. Lower your heels back down, and you have just completed one repetition (see Figure 9). Continue with the exercise until your calf muscles start to feel some exhaustion. Then stop to rest. That is one set. The capacity for the calves to perform isolated strength training like this varies greatly from person to person. For you, this may range from 5 repetitions up to 35, or maybe more. Just complete one set while getting used to this routine early on. After a couple of weeks of doing the exercise, add a second set.

Once you build up adequate strength, you can perform the exercise while holding a pair of dumbbells to provide greater resistance. Or, just do more repetitions. Either way builds both strength and endurance; a routine with more weight and less repetitions sides toward strength building, less weight with more repetitions emphasizes endurance. Both are beneficial.

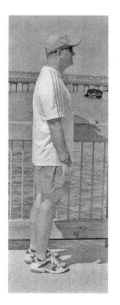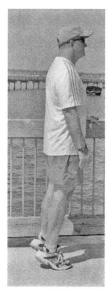

Figure 9: Standing calf raise starting position (left picture) and flexed position (right picture)

Seated Calf Raise

Here you pretty much need to use additional resistance, as you'll be seated and your body weight won't help you work out the calf muscles. Take a seat with your feet resting flat directly in front of you, legs bent at a 90-degree angle, keeping your knees directly above your heels. Place a towel or padding of some kind across your knees. On top of the towel or padding place a weight, a barbell plate for instance, and simply raise your heels up off the ground (see Figure 10) similar to how you did in the standing calf raise. Keep completing the motion until exhaustion sets in, and then stop. Just complete one set with this exercise as well. Add another set or two later if and when you feel ready.

If you don't have a barbell plate handy, you could use a different form of resistance, such as a pair of phone books. Or, you could actually push down on your knees with the palms of your hands, supplying the resistance with your upper body strength. Your imagination is the only limit here.

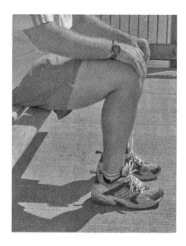 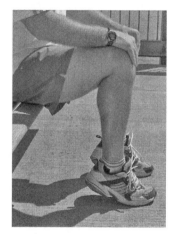

Figure 10: Seated calf raise starting position (left picture) and flexed position (right picture)

After performing these exercises, remember to stretch the muscles you just worked. (See Chapter 8 for calf stretches.)

These are not complicated exercises, nor are they very exciting. But they get the job done. It's pretty much a matter of buckling down and grinding out the repetitions. Remember, it takes a while to adapt to strength training. You may get sore a day or two after the first couple of times you specifically work out your calves, so don't overdo it. At the same time, don't worry too much if a little soreness does occur. Of all the muscles in the body, the calf is one of the most resilient. It is used pretty much every day if a person walks at all, and is thus designed for plenty of rigor. So you can work the calves hard and with regularity, every other day or so being ideal. Do this consistently and your calf muscles will serve as a better support system for your recuperating feet.

16

Strengthen Your Arches

In addition to working on your flexibility, you'll want to build strength in the arch of your foot. Flimsy muscles in this area will leave your plantar fascia at continued risk, whereas strong ones will stabilize and protect it. The arch controls the impact experienced when walking or running, and stabilizes the foot while standing in place. So the stronger your arch is the better.

Strong arch muscles will not only help you heal from plantar fasciitis sooner, they will guard against its recurrence. Preventing recurrence is no small matter when talking about plantar fasciitis; it is a condition that tends to sneak back into the picture if you're not careful.

Fortunately, developing strength in the arch of your foot is not hard. Sometimes, it's actually kind of fun. You just have to make a habit of it. See the following pair of exercises for some easy yet valuable arch strengthening. Do both of them while seated in a comfortable chair.

Towel Scrunch

Place a towel on the floor in front of you. Use just your toes to drag or "scrunch" the towel toward you (see Figure 11). You should be able to feel the muscles in your arch really flex. Success is attained when you've scrunched the entire towel into a bunch. Repeat the action again. Do this every other day, and try to work up to about 8 or 10 repetitions over time. (Note: you'll find it easier to do the towel scrunch on a smooth surface; carpet can provide quite the resistance when using a terry-cloth towel.)

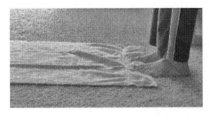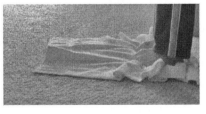

Figure 11: Towel scrunch starting position (left picture) and during the scrunching (right picture)

Coin pickup

For the coin pickup, simply set out some coins at your feet instead of a towel. Then grab a coin under or between a couple of your toes (see Figure 12). Do this with different toe combinations, allowing each toe to get in on the action. Set the grasped coins off to one side, until you've made a separate pile with them. Then go ahead and move the coins in a similar manner with your other foot. Do this exercise every other day.

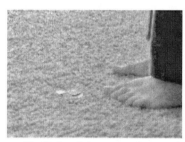 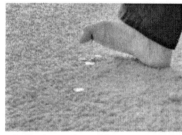

Figure 12: Coin pickup starting position (left picture) and in-process position (right picture)

Do the coin pickup on the same day you perform the towel scrunch. This will work out your arch muscles thoroughly and from different angles, and then allow them a day to recover and regenerate in a little better shape than before. The rest day is especially important when you are just starting this foot strengthening routine. It will let your foot adjust and adapt to the targeted exercises. Also remember to gently stretch your arch after performing these exercises (see Chapter 9).

That's all there is to it. The towel scrunch and the coin pickup exercises are really convenient. You can do them even while reading or watching TV. And they are effective as well. You should feel the muscles working as you carry out the exercises and maybe some soreness the next day when you're just getting started.

Even though the exercises may be fun, or even feel funny for that matter, know that you are accomplishing some serious strength training at the same time. Coupled with a durable, supportive pair of shoes, stronger arch muscles will help get your feet back in good stead.

17

Strengthen Your Abdominals

The benefits of strong abdominals are many, not the least of which is better posture. Strong abdominals support the spine's normal curvature, stabilize the trunk, allow better control of your leg movements, and encourage better foot motion when walking and running. The reinforcement realized in the curvature of your back from strong abdominal muscles will reduce the compression forces on your spine when you walk and run. This will keep your back safe, and consequently you'll be less likely to alter your good stride to compensate for a sore lower back. And in your body's long chain of biomechanical events, the better leg movements and controlled foot strike will lessen the wear and tear on your feet.

Numerous abdominal exercises exist, and here are three of them. Performing all three should provide a well-rounded workout to the three primary areas of the abdominals: upper abdominals, lower abdominals, and the obliques (those muscles on the sides of your abdominal area).

Crunch

The crunch works your upper abdominals. Lie on your back with your knees bent, feet resting on the floor. Put your hands across your chest. Slowly curl up and lift your shoulder blades off the floor (see Figure 13). Hold for three seconds and lower yourself slowly. Repeat this just a few times if you're new to abdominal work. Eventually your total repetitions could increase; you may work up to 20, 30, 40, or more. But for now do just 5-10 repetitions.

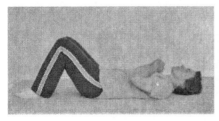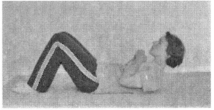

Figure 13: Crunch starting position (left picture) and flexed position (right picture)

Knee raise

The knee raise works your lower abdominals. Continue to lie on your back, with your knees bent, feet resting on the floor, and your hands at your sides or across your chest. Slowly pull your knees up and toward your chest (see Figure 14). At the point where you feel your abdominals flex, hold that position for three seconds or so, then lower your feet back to the floor. Like the crunch, repeat the knee raise just a handful of times, maybe 5-10 repetitions. With time you may work up to 20 or more.

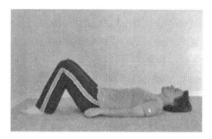 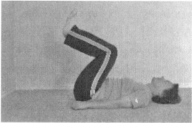

Figure 14: Knee raise starting position (left picture) and flexed position (right picture)

Standing Twist

The standing twist works your obliques. Hold an unweighted bar, broom handle, dowel rod, or walking stick across your shoulders, or just place your hands behind your head. Stand with your knees slightly bent. While keeping your hips stationary, twist slowly to the left, hold for about three seconds, then to the right, and again hold the position (see Figure 15). Avoid swinging your hips as you twist.

The twist is not as intense as the crunch or the knee raise motions, so you may be able to do more repetitions comfortably. Try 20 at first. Work up to more repetitions over time.

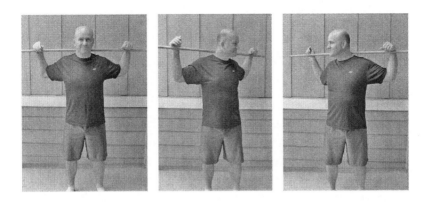

Figure 15: Standing twist starting illustration (left picture), twisting to the left (middle picture) and twisting to the right (right picture)

18

Stay Well-Hydrated

Hydration is often overlooked as a major factor in injury recovery. But replenishing your body with plenty of water and other nutritious fluids will give your plantar fasciitis recuperation a boost. Staying well-hydrated is very important to your overall health; if you're chronically dehydrated, plantar fasciitis may represent just one of your worries.

Maintaining ideal hydration benefits your digestion, skin, hair, brain function, strength, and endurance. Adequate hydration will help ward off colds and flu. It will assist in heart health. If a person's hydration level drops even 5%, metabolism can slow as much as 30%. So any weight maintenance or weight loss efforts will be far easier with regular water intake (which in turn will help you heal from plantar fasciitis: lower body weight = less plantar fascia strain).

When you become dehydrated, so do your ligaments, muscles, and tendons. Connective tissue in the human body depends on water for elasticity and stability. Muscle function, including that of your calf and foot muscles, will be diminished with lack of hydration. This is exacerbated as your body's blood volume is reduced, or in other words, when the oxygen reaching the muscles becomes limited. Muscle performance will further suffer. This means weakening, tightness, and possible cramping. More strain on your plantar fascia will result.

So make a conscious effort to consume plenty of fluids each day. And drink before you get thirsty. Under normal circumstances, with normal food intake, that fluid should be primarily water. Drink about 5-8 glasses of water a day. However, the water content in liquids like milk, orange juice, hot cocoa, and vegetable juice does count toward this total. Water contained in alcohol and in caffeinated drinks like cola and coffee do not, due to the diuretic effect these beverages have on the body.

Of course, it's best to do all things in moderation. When replacing lost fluids, there is no need to drink a gallon of water in a sitting. Try to rehydrate with the approximate amount of water you lost over time, whether through normal activities or through vigorous work or exercise. If you are exercising heavily or enduring hot weather, in either case sweating profusely, you may want to consume a commercial sport drink to replace potassium, sodium, and other electrolytes at the same time that you rehydrate. This option is more effective for rejuvenation than plain water when fluid loss has been great, as described above. And it will help you avoid a condition known as hyponatremia, defined by a dangerously low concentration of sodium in the blood.

Hyponatremia results when heavy water loss takes place, and the only fluid replacement you provide for your body is water alone, especially a large amount of water, which can cause the level of bloodstream minerals to drop. When mineral levels in your blood are low, such as sodium, water in your bloodstream may move into your brain, where concentrations of sodium are higher. This process is the normal attempt of human physiology to even things out. In this case, however, it can be bad news. The pressure in your brain could increase, and at the very least cause dizziness. It can also cause twitches, stupor, seizures, unconsciousness, and brain damage. So use good judgment when drinking back on lost fluids. Don't worry, an extra glass of water will not do this. A few extra glasses of plain water might though, if consumed all at once while you're dehydrated. When seeking replenishment, include some nutritious foods along with water, especially those which contain potassium and sodium. Or as mentioned, consume a commercial sport drink, which has been designed to replace the lost minerals.

In summary, be sensible when rehydrating. But by all means, make sure you take the time and effort to do it. Plan ahead and have drinks on hand before, during and after exercise, throughout your work days, and on outings of any kind. Adequate hydration can serve as a substantial aid in your healing process.

19

Massage Your Feet By Hand

Applying a massage to your feet by hand will assist your body in removing waste products and jump-start healing. A massage by hand allows you to customize the pressure and location of the massage with great specificity. But do this carefully. You may be tempted to really dig your fingers and thumbs in with extra force, but go easy. Remember, there's not an evil life form in there that you are trying to crush. You are kneading the tissues of your injured foot. Therefore, tender loving care is the order of the day. Very forceful pressure could worsen the condition, as the injured portion of the foot is already inflamed.

Proponents of massage believe that it encourages healing by manipulating the tissue at hand, and in so doing, promotes relaxation, better blood flow, and the elimination of waste products. And in the case of plantar fasciitis, massage can serve to break up scar tissue which is forming and allow the injured tissue to heal faster.

The actual technique for self-massaging your feet is simple. Just rest one foot across your opposite knee, and with both hands palpitate the underside of the foot from the base of your toes all the way to the back your heel. Do this for a few minutes, and feel the result. If certain spots trigger sharp pain, for instance the area at the front of the heel, discontinue the massage, at least for the time being. You may benefit from the same action in the future, maybe in a few weeks once your healing has progressed. Or, perhaps massage will not be the best thing for your particular condition, in which case you should discontinue it. But you won't know until you try it a time or two.

You may, on the other hand, experience significant relief immediately. You'll have to feel the situation out, no pun intended. If gentle massage does give you immediate relief, do it regularly as part of your regimen. Once a day is not too often. This convenient procedure may do the trick to erase soreness, clear out waste products in the tissues of your foot, and quicken your recovery. It may also diminish the return of pain as you resume activity. And, hey, sometimes it just feels good!

20

Roll with It

This next activity will keep the progress of your foot recovery rolling, literally. Rolling with a tennis ball, that is. Sit in your favorite chair, place a tennis ball on the floor in front of you, and gently roll it back and forth underneath the length of your foot. This is yet another way to massage your injured area, with a slightly different approach than a massage by hand. Like massaging your feet by hand, rolling the foot atop a tennis ball breaks up adhesions which are forming on the traumatized tissue, and allows a more complete and rapid healing process to take place. Blood flow will be improved as well, helping to whisk away waste materials, further assisting your injury in a quicker repair.

As an alternative to the tennis ball, use an ice-filled plastic bottle. The bottles used for 16- and 20-ounce sport drinks and soft drinks work well. Just fill one about ¾ full with water and place it in the freezer for a few hours. Then it should be ready to go. Proceed as you did with the tennis ball. Remember to either wear socks or place a towel over the bottle so there's a protective layer between your skin and the ice; you don't want frost bite, after all!

When rolling your ailing feet atop an ice bottle, you're doing double duty for them: a stimulating massage coupled with an ice treatment. Take it easy in terms of pressure applied with an ice bottle, as compared to a tennis ball. Whereas the tennis ball has a little give, the bottle will be solid. Don't press too hard and make your already injured foot tissue more so.

Also, if you've just iced your feet, you may opt to use just the tennis ball, instead of an ice bottle. You don't want to ice an injury to excess, so limit ice to 10 to 15 minutes a day at the most. If you have not yet iced your feet on a given day, keep the ice bottle option in mind for quick relief. It fulfills ice and massage therapy at the same time.

21

Massage Your Calf Muscles

Just as flexible, pliable calf muscles reduce the tension on the plantar fascia, relaxed ones will have the same effect. You can ease the tension and help this set of muscles relax with massage. The more the entire calf area is relieved of tightness and soreness, the less strain that your heel will undergo.

Remember the analogy of the archer's bow as it relates to calf tightness and strain on the plantar fascia. When the calf lacks flexibility, it's as if the bow limbs are pulling on the string with undue force. Apply massage to the calf area to help ease the tension on the "bow limbs."

Feel free to massage your calf muscles with more vigor than you did your feet. Within the realm of plantar fasciitis, the calf muscles are not injured, unlike your feet. Therefore, a bit more force can be put to work here without harm. Other than that, the procedure for this self-massage is similar to that used for the feet. Sections of muscle where you feel soreness from working on your feet or exercising will be obvious, but massage the whole area, from the larger top section of the calf down to just above the heel area.

An additional benefit you will reap from a calf massage routine is the accelerated removal of waste products from the tissues, thereby gaining quicker recovery from any strength training or exercise you may have performed. You'll get stronger calf muscles in less time; strength gained in the calf area is always a boon to the solid foundation needed to recover from plantar fasciitis, as well as ward off its return. So dig in.

22

Tighten Your Shoes

Supportive, well-fitting shoes can only do their job if the material of which they are composed fits the contours of your foot. Just as you should not wear shoes that are too big, you are better off if you don't leave shoes, even those with a proper fit, too loose on your feet. It may seem that since plantar fasciitis has set in and you are battling the resulting inflammation, the looser the footwear the better. On the contrary; loose shoes can immensely irritate your injury. I found this through trial and error. At times, soreness would return unexpectedly when walking. I couldn't believe the difference it made when I tied any of the shoes I wore just a little tighter. Often the soreness creeping up in my heel would be reduced, and other times it would disappear completely.

Think snug here, not constricting. Certainly don't crank down and form a tourniquet with your laces. You just want each shoe to hug your foot a bit and not slide all over with each step. You may need to do some experimentation here. At times, you might secure the laces too tight, and have to readjust them after a few steps. And if you are on a lengthy walk or standing for a long time, your feet may normally and naturally swell a little. This could also require an adjustment in your shoes' tightness. It might seem like a bother having to fiddle over and over with your shoes, but once you get them secured just right you'll see what I mean. The shape and construction of the shoes are then allowed to support your arch, cushion your landing, and control the motion of your feet. You'll find yourself stepping along easier and with less discomfort.

If you stop to rest, or you're going to be sitting for a while, by all means loosen the shoes for that period of time. Blood flow and relaxation will be at their optimum when shoes are loose. Let your circulation work in the best environment possible. Tighten the shoes back down when you get back up to walk, though. Sound like too much trouble? It can get annoying...but, these are your feet we're talking about here. It's all part of the adjustments you make when recovering from plantar fasciitis. Go to the extra trouble to snug your shoes to their optimum fit, and let them protect your feet in the manner for which they were designed.

23

Elevate Your Feet

Any chance you get to elevate your feet, do so. Elevating them will enhance blood flow and aid in the removal of waste products from the injury. Elevation reduces the blood pressure in the area and thus the swelling. Additionally, the improved circulation will allow better delivery of nutrients to the injured tissue, helping the tissue to heal. Your recovery process will speed up as a result.

You basically want to elevate your feet above the level of your heart. Nothing too scientific here. The most practical way to do this is to simply lie on your back and prop your feet up. You can use a couple of pillows, or maybe even the arm rest of a couch or a cushioned chair.

Try to elevate the feet for 10-20 minutes. If you can only fit in 5 minutes or so at a given time, still treat yourself to it. Elevation of the feet is a course of action where you can feel the relief immediately. Especially if you've just been on your feet for a long time or you've been out walking or running. Once you do it a time or two, you'll probably need no further encouragement. Your feet will feel noticeable relief. Not to mention, the session might give you a chance to unwind, read, or rest, so the benefits of powering down to prop up your feet may be multiple.

Whoever thought doing so little could do so much? Keep this effortless tactic in mind and use it to expedite your progress back to healthier feet. All while you lie down, stretch out, and relax.

24

Maintain Low Impact Form

In addition to becoming stronger and more flexible, you'll want to minimize one of the primary enemies of your feet: impact. Here are some ways to do that.

Shorten your stride, whether walking, running, or just moving about. Changing the length with which you step can seem awkward at first, but a short time after consciously adjusting your stride you'll most likely stick to it for good. A short stride feels more efficient and actually helps you move forward faster. It will feel better on your feet and heels. And it will decrease your chance of an additional cumulative stress injury.

A heavy heel strike results from a long, reaching stride. More impact on your feet is the outcome. A lengthy stride can result in more soreness in your knees, hamstrings, quadriceps, and shins. It is inefficient and actually wastes energy. And the added impact will be brutal on your feet. This can really add up if you run, as running produces impact at least several times your body weight, even up to 10 times. Although the stress will be realized more intensely if you run, the force upon your feet can be about 1.5 times your body weight even when walking. As opposed to a long, lumbering stride, a shorter stride benefits you when walking also, since it helps minimize the force upon your feet.

Besides using a shorter stride, practice an ideal foot strike. When either walking or running, you may find it tempting to land on the balls of your feet, or even on your tiptoes. It would stand to reason, since sharp pain emanates from your heels, to keep contact with the ground as far from your heels as possible. However, you should avoid this urge. When you land on the balls of your feet or your tiptoes, you actually stress the plantar fascia *more*, not less. The stress realized during any long walks or distance running while landing on your tiptoes will be felt immediately. And it won't feel pleasant.

Similarly, you should avoid walking or running on the outside edges of your feet. This type of foot placement will not let the foot roll forward as it was meant to, and like landing on your tiptoes, will probably compound your injury.

You should still land on your heel with each step – ideally toward the *front* of the heel, right around the middle of the foot. Landing on the middle of the foot goes along with a shorter, controlled stride, and results in better shock absorption. You avoid the excessive force from a strike at the very back of the heel, which is all but impossible to avoid if your stride is more like a long, exaggerated lunge.

Even if you feel a little soreness, let the foot roll forward as it does during non-injured walking and running. Landing with the middle of the foot will assist with an ideal rolling forward motion. And remember, good shoes should protect the injured area of your feet to a large extent. So again, make sure you wear good shoes.

And finally, glide with your feet, don't thump. Let your feet float just above the ground with each step. Don't raise way up and pound the foot down with each step. If you're one of the countless people who walk and run like this (I myself was one), now is the time to adjust the forceful landing you inflict upon your feet.

I know of what I speak here, as I was one of the greatest offenders. For years, I would bound along when running, reaching as far as I could with each leg. My lead foot would fly way above the ground, and then crash down upon landing. My legs and feet would take a terrible pounding, but I persisted with this self-defeating stride. I actually trained for and ran numerous 8K and 10K races this way. In fact, during downhill sections of some courses, I would leap up and out as much as possible with each step, letting myself become airborne for a moment before crushing impact met each footfall. I figured, why not just let gravity take me? And I wondered why my shins were on fire and my hamstring muscles almost nonfunctional with soreness for days afterward. Not to mention, it seemed like the runners whom I had burst past on the downhill portion, the ones with more relaxed, controlled strides, always seemed to pass me up a short time later. It took a painful bout of plantar fasciitis to step back and examine what I was doing wrong.

Having trouble picturing what I mean here? If you've ever watched a major league baseball game, and saw the defenders make a key third out, or better yet a double play to end the inning, you may have seen the players then proudly bound off the field. Way up, way down, loping along with vitality, thundering down with each step of their heroic all-star jog. It looks impressive, and it's actually kind of fun to run that way. But if your feet are in the process of healing, restrain yourself. Looking good and feeling good can be two different things. Go easy on your legs, protect your knees, and be kind to your feet. Keep your stride short. Make contact with the front of your heel, or your midfoot. Keep your feet low to the ground, whisking them along and planting them quickly but gently. You'll walk and run with more efficiency, move just as fast if not faster than before, and expose your body to far less damaging impact.

25

Avoid Dangerous Surfaces and Limit Steep Hills

Be careful where you walk and run. Some hazards are obvious. Others can disguise themselves better, and may even look inviting.

Icy areas represent probably the most evident example of a dangerous surface. With your feet slipping, sliding, gliding, and floating unpredictably in any direction, icy surfaces can inflict extra damage to your already tender plantar fascia. And on those flat icy areas with ice and snow chunks frozen in place, walking can be horrific. Don't attempt to navigate ice-covered areas unless you absolutely have to.

Moving across any type of surface which is uneven will be questionable to the safety of your feet. Luckily, walking in such an area will feel uncomfortable, and you'd probably sense that it's not good for your feet. And you'd be right. The foot in the lower position is subject to undue stress, as it carries an excessive proportion of the load in this situation. Choose relatively even surfaces if you can.

But what about a nice sandy beach, or the local park's big, green expanse of grass? Absolutely lovely settings, right? Proceed with caution. Both of these surfaces can actually stress the plantar fascia to a great degree. Walking or running in soft, sandy areas can be deceptively rough on your feet. Trudging in the sand will often result in the heel plunging below the level of the forefoot at the moment your weight comes to bear over your entire foot. While the heel is in this negative position, it experiences far more pressure than when walking on level ground: the additional force can actually be three or four times greater. A sandy surface may look alluring, but watch out.

Grassy areas pose a mixed scenario: grass has some positive aspects and some negative ones too. The cushion grass provides is undeniable, and it's definitely a good thing. Not much brutal impact will be realized on grass. On the other hand, lawns and fields of grass are inevitably uneven. Bumps, dips, pieces of litter, roots, and rocks can lie hidden anywhere in grass, as can actual holes made by rodents. So despite the padding grass provides, it is not an optimum surface on which to walk or run when recovering from plantar fasciitis.

And of course, we all know the reality of unyielding concrete, as that's what most sidewalks consist of. Concrete is unforgiving, absorbing almost no shock from your footfalls. Much better choices for walking are dirt, gravel or wood chip paths, providing they are even and in good condition. Asphalt is actually not a bad surface either, specifically in warm weather. It becomes somewhat shock-absorbing as the sun heats it and makes it soft. In extreme cold, however, it becomes as unforgiving as concrete.

Beware of hills as well. Like grassy surfaces, traveling on hills contains desirable and not so desirable aspects. The vigorous climbs and descents steep hills provide can build strength, endurance, and muscle tone to a great degree, especially in the very leg muscles you need to solidify for future injury protection. However, when traveling uphill, the ankle is forced into what is called *dorsiflexion*. Dorsiflexion means the foot bends back so your toes are closer to your shin. While in this position, the plantar fascia is getting stretched, and in some cases strained, as it bears the weight of the rest of your body being heaved up the hill. On the downhill trip, the ankle goes into the opposite position, *plantar flexion*. The plantar flexion position results in a similar foot strike as when walking on the balls of your feet, which is detrimental to the feet at any time, but especially when recovering from plantar fasciitis. Add to the fact that your body weight is pounding down with extra momentum thanks to gravity on your downhill descent, and the result is a significant load for your injured feet to bear. Walking and especially running on hills can be rough on a plantar fasciitis sufferer.

Is there any way to limit the strain from traveling up and down hills? I found one strategy helps above all else: keep your stride short. Don't reach way up when going uphill. And don't step big and allow your weight to crash down on your leading foot on the downhill descent. Landing on your midfoot will help also, as it keeps your foot more level, and diminishes the extreme positions of dorsiflexion and plantar flexion. If you keep your stride short, striking on the midfoot is much easier to accomplish.

Are you expected to maneuver on completely flat and perfectly forgiving surfaces at all times? Of course not. That would be difficult if not impossible to achieve as you move through your day or go for walks in various areas. Hard or slippery surfaces, small hills, and short but steep inclines occur in most areas, and you can travel on them to a limited extent without a problem. The key to remember is the concept of *cumulative stress*. Plantar fasciitis results because of stress, strain, wear and tear occurring over and over from certain damaging factors. Try to avoid risky areas and steep hills if you can, and certainly don't plan to exercise on them.

26

Experiment with Heel Cups and Arch Supports

You may want to supplement your new, robust, highly-protective shoes with one of a couple of types of orthotic inserts. Heel cups and arch supports are easily acquired and surprisingly helpful for some people. They can relieve discomfort, promote healing, and ward off a recurrence of plantar fasciitis.

A heel cup is simply an insert that is placed in the back of your shoe, to add cushioning and lift your heel a bit. The human foot is equipped with a padding of fat covering the heel. This padding protects your foot against impact and wear. With time, rigor, and age, however, the padding begins to spread out, and some of its shock-absorbing effectiveness is lost. A heel cup will help compensate for this diminished natural protection. It may also supply some cushioning which a given pair of shoes does not have.

Like the heel cup, arch supports can compensate for natural protection that your foot lacks, or for a shortcoming in a particular pair of shoes you're wearing. An arch support will help prevent your plantar fascia from excessive stretching. When your arches collapse or sag, they tug against the fascia's point of attachment on your heel. The arch support will help alleviate this. If your experience is anything like mine, you'll feel immediate relief once you put a pair of arch supports to use.

Heel cups and arch supports can be purchased over-the-counter, and most every footwear dealer, pharmacy and department store seems to carry at least one brand. Your best bet is to visit a running, walking, or other specialty store relating to fitness. Such stores will have the best selection, often with a knowledgeable staff to help you.

Heel cups and arch supports may help a little or help a lot. Very little risk is involved in experimenting with either. The tightness of your shoes may need to be adjusted after adding either a heel cup or an arch support. You may want to loosen the laces a bit to accommodate the new protective layer in your shoes. Other than that, place either type of insert in your shoes, and you're ready to go. Give heel cups or arch supports, or both, a try. They are inexpensive and can provide surprising relief for such simple devices. See what you think. They just might bolster the natural protection your body provides, and help you heal faster while preventing foot pain.

27

Consume Plenty of Antioxidants

To keep your body's healing powers on overdrive, fortify yourself with a regular dose of antioxidants. Your body already helps protect itself by producing certain enzymes which serve as antioxidants. You can add to this protection by consuming antioxidant-rich foods.

What purpose do antioxidants serve? The physiological process of oxidation occurs normally as part of your body's functioning, such as in respiration and metabolism. However, oxidation also produces the deleterious byproducts known as "free radical" molecules. The incidence of physical exertion, injury, and stress will increase the normal quantity of free radicals, and they will then accumulate more quickly. If their presence becomes too great, they can cause cell damage, which is part of the "oxidative stress" process. This process can bring about several negative consequences, among which is the slowing of your body's ability to heal.

Perhaps the most dramatic benefit of antioxidants in your diet is their conquest over oxidants, i.e., free radicals. Antioxidants detect and scavenge these unwanted free radicals. The free radicals are then neutralized and eliminated. As a consequence, antioxidants reduce inflammation, which improves circulation. Tissue damage will be minimized; damaged tissue will be more quickly repaired. And healing will be thus accelerated. In a similar fashion, you will recover from workouts and strengthening exercises more easily. Consequently you'll become stronger that much faster.

As a nice side benefit, those foods which contain lots of antioxidants also tend to be highly nutritious. Mind and body will function better in every way when your nutrition level is tip-top. You'll feel fully operational with fewer calories when you supply yourself with high-nutrient fuel. What's more, antioxidants allow your system to better utilize nutrients you've consumed. You'll get more "bang for the bite" from the food components you eat.

How can you make sure your normal diet includes enough antioxidants? To simplify matters, if you regularly eat fruits and vegetables, you will get at least a fair supply of antioxidants. So make sure you do. To really boost your system's recuperative abilities, check out the following list of antioxidant top performers. Include some or all of them as part of your regular eating routine.

Excellent antioxidant sources:
Blueberries, strawberries, cherries, apples, grapes, cranberries, raspberries, blackberries, olives, seeds, peanuts, walnuts, almonds, avocado, whole wheat, beans, broccoli, seafood, beef, pork, chicken, brown rice, cantaloupe, peppers, spinach, squash, sweet potatoes, and citrus fruit.

In addition, black and green teas are loaded with antioxidants, so if you already enjoy either of these, continue drinking them. And good news for coffee drinkers: recent studies have found coffee, both regular and decaf, to be loaded with antioxidants. Yay!

Some other interesting antioxidant sources are red wine, dark chocolate, and honey. This does not necessarily mean you should gobble down a whole chocolate bar, eat a jar of honey, and wash it down with an entire bottle of wine. Moderation in all things. Think sips and morsels when it comes to these very sweet items.

You'll want to partake of antioxidant-rich foods as part of your plantar fasciitis recovery process, to be sure. But really, eating such foods is a good habit to get into for life. Your feet will heal quicker, but also, a high antioxidant intake will help ward off illness and just plain make you feel better. Get into the routine of consuming food which contains plenty of antioxidants, and your injury recovery program and overall health will take a big step forward.

28

Track Your Food Intake

There is no getting around it: a lower body weight will mean less strain on your feet. If you carry a little extra weight, and many of us do, now is the time to commit to reducing some of that excess. Just a few less pounds on your frame can result in significant relief to your injured feet.

But I must mention: as with any weight loss program, consult a physician, especially if you're already under the care of one and/or have special dietary needs or restrictions. If not consulting a physician, follow government guidelines as to what constitutes a healthy weight for you. DO NOT think you need to lose weight to heal from plantar fasciitis. That said, this chapter only applies to you if you actually have excess weight to lose. If you're at an already appropriate weight, skip this chapter.

Reams of books have been written on weight loss. This book is not one of them. I will not turn this into a weight loss seminar, but at the same time, I'd be derelict in my duties if I failed to mention the subject of body weight while discussing plantar fasciitis recovery. And I won't just blurt out "Lose weight." That would oversimplify a very complex issue. For many folks, weight control is a life-long challenge. And that includes me.

So I'll propose one course of action that you can try. It is the least original advice you may have ever heard. It's old advice. In fact, it's almost worn out advice. But it's the type of advice that, if followed, always pays off.

Write down each and every thing you eat in a given day.

Doesn't sound too profound or exciting, does it? But…when was the last time you did it? If you choose to follow this advice, I think you will find three things:

- You're probably eating more than you think.
- You're letting less-than-desirable foods sneak into your daily intake.
- You're able to eat plenty, actually indulge yourself, if you cut the diabolical but always available junk food from your diet.

And if your experience is anything like mine, you'll skip a lot of bad food choices when you're faced with writing each one down.

Keep the recording of your intake basic for best results. You'll want an uncomplicated system in order to keep with it for a sustained time period. Not to mention, to start doing it in the first place. Perhaps use a pocket-sized calendar or even a post-it or two during the day. Then copy it down later into a log, using something as simple as a notebook or a tablet.

Find a nutrition book which lists calorie counts, or bookmark one of the numerous websites out there which contain the information. Then track the associated calories of each item. Don't have access to these resources, and don't know the calorie count on a given item? Guess at it. You can look it up later. The important thing is to list the item and help yourself become aware of what you are eating. (Of course, record what you drink each day also. Many calories can slip in quickly through beverages if you let them.)

Soon you'll get the system down and the calorie counts memorized. After the first few days, try to winnow down the calories slightly. Maybe reduce them 5% or so, 10% at the most. Change your eating habits slowly but steadily. Try this regimen for just two weeks. You may be surprised at what you find, and at the results you experience. If you like what you see, stick with it for another week or two.

Logging what you eat each day will not only help you monitor how much you take in, it will also help you track the *types* of calories you consume. This leads me to qualify the statement made above regarding bodyweight as it relates to plantar fasciitis. A heavier body due to lots of muscle will in fact subject your feet to a little more stress than a lighter body would. But keep the muscle. It's too important as a fat burner to lose it. Muscle on your frame boosts the quietly purring furnace of your metabolism a bit; you will burn extra calories just maintaining the muscle. Healthier food choices allow you to maintain the muscle that much easier. And, happily, lower your body fat percentage instead.

So, what exactly should you eat on a regular basis for best results? This is an enormous subject, but perhaps it's best to begin with what you should *not* eat. Extensive studies, journals, and textbooks have been completed on the subject of nutrition. But as for foods to avoid, you knew most of the answers back in grade school. Here are just a few obvious examples of items to limit or completely avoid: donuts, cheese puffs, pre-wrapped snack cakes, apple fritters, super-sized fries, fast food hamburgers and hotdogs made with fiber-free white buns, most types of candy, and cream-filled long johns. Just to name a few.

Am I making your mouth water? Sorry. But I think you get the picture. And I bet you already knew the items mentioned were ill-advised. The stuff is tempting though, isn't it? And it's so readily available nowadays. To help you dig your heels in and resist temptations like these, start writing them down when you snack on any.

You will find that when diligently tracking your intake, the notion of notating down the record of a gooey snack item, which took you maybe two minutes total to eat, then jotting a whopping 400, 500, or 600 as the calorie value, will in fact be daunting. You will start to think twice about such transgressions if you hold yourself accountable in writing. Tracking your intake will help you form better eating habits.

What can you replace these questionable goodies with? I'm not a nutritionist, but after researching the subject for myself, I found some things that work for me. Here are my suggestions.

Fruits and vegetables should represent a mainstay in your diet. No surprise there. But once you wean yourself off sweet snacks filled with refined sugar, you might not believe how sweet and satisfying a piece of fruit tastes. Try it for awhile. Barring any allergies to them, include a variety of nuts in your diet. Not only are nuts convenient snacks, but they contain large amounts of protein and heart-healthy fats. Switch from whole milk to 1% or skim. Replace white bread, noodles, and rice with whole grain varieties. You'll get full sooner and stay satisfied much longer.

Avoid any product which contains hydrogenated oils, also called "trans fats." Trans fats are oils artificially processed for longer storage; they are unnatural, of little food value, and hard on your cardiovascular system. For good sources of fats, turn to oils such as safflower and olive oils. Like nuts, they contain the kind of healthy fats you want in your diet. Lean meats are good in moderation. Trim and discard any extra fat on the cuts as well as the skin on poultry. Eat fish, from freshwater or the ocean, on a regular basis. Fish are low in calories, packed with protein, and certain types, especially salmon and trout, serve as a source of healthful fats.

For a sweetener, it's hard to beat honey. Honey digests slower than table sugar, so you avoid the quick surge and crash often associated with sweet foods. Honey contains antioxidants, and is sweet enough to satisfy those desperate cravings a person gets from time to time. If you long for candy, and can't hold back, opt for chocolate. Choose dark chocolate if it's available. It too contains antioxidants. And the intense flavor of dark chocolate should stop a sweet tooth in its tracks. Chocolate has lots of calories though, so limit the portions you imbibe in.

Don't obsess over losing weight. Track your food intake, keep exercising, and see where you can substitute better foods for the high-calorie, low-value ones. Whatever happens, happens. Even if you don't lose an ounce, your system will be fortified with higher quality nutrients with which to repair your injured feet.

Tracking your food intake daily almost guarantees you'll eat a little less, and the foods you do eat will be healthier. And you may lose some weight in the process. Your recovering feet will then have less of a load to bear.

29

Avoid Jumping Back In Too Soon

Recovery from a bout with plantar fasciitis is quite the balancing act, isn't it? You must strategically restrain yourself from harmful activities, giving yourself a break from the source of your injury. Yet, experts generally agree that exercise and strengthening are not only OK but required for recovery. So far you've been encouraged to stretch, strengthen, move, and eat better. After all that, you must feel ready to get back into the action. Maybe with even more vigor than before.

Not so fast. In addition to all its other annoying aspects, plantar fasciitis has a nasty habit of recurring. So proceed with caution.

Remember, nurture your body, not your pride.

For instance, if you were able to make special arrangements at a job to accommodate your condition, see if you can transition back into your normal duties little by little. Don't declare full recovery too quickly. Work back into the groove slowly over time.

When it comes to walking for exercise, push yourself a little, but remember to rein your enthusiasm in at the same time. Especially if you feel really revved up, as in trying to break your old records by a long shot. Walking is low impact and therefore pretty ideal as a recovery activity, but it can be overdone just like anything else. Enjoy in moderation.

If you are a runner, start back up with very conservative durations and speed. Forget what you used to do in terms of time and distance. The same goes for bicycling. And even more so for high action, stop-and-go activities like tennis. When transitioning back into the "old you," you need to do it gradually. Be enthused, but don't erase your recent progress with extreme enthusiasm that turns out to be your undoing.

Maybe rearrange your goals from what they were previously. Don't think of this as setting your sights lower; think of it as taking care of yourself. I'd say the fact that you can get back into endeavors like running, biking, or tennis at all is its own victory. Same with resuming walking, hiking, and other sports you love. Have fun, but not too much fun!

And, it should be said, keep on with your recovery exercises. Continue to stretch every day. Do the strengthening exercises on a regular basis. More flexible and stronger arches and calf muscles will only continue to help you. Make sure to eat good, healthy food and avoid unhealthy food. Don't eat huge quantities of either. Make these positive actions part of your daily routine.

Ease back into things. However humble your progress is at first, remember that you're making a comeback; enjoy the excitement and accomplishment that goes along with it.

30

Visualize Success and Move On

Since beginning your battle with plantar fasciitis, how do you see yourself? As an invalid? Or as a bundle of strength and energy, stymied by a physical setback just for the moment? Do you picture never-ending misery from your foot pain, or success and healthy feet right around the corner?

I believe the difference between a negative and a positive attitude, and thus the self image you maintain, can lead to very different results as you try to recuperate from plantar fasciitis. A positive attitude can serve as a major factor in a speedy recovery process. In a similar way, so can your self-image as it relates to your injury.

The body and mind are unquestionably linked. Ever had a tension headache? Most people have. If and when you've had one, do you recall anyone clamping a big vice on your head and tightening it down? Or were you hit on the head with a rubber mallet just before the headache hit? Probably not. Most likely, the headache was caused by what you perceived about the events happening around you; events that were frustrating and helped you get stressed out. What went on in your mind led to a quite tangible tension headache. Your mind and body can be very closely linked. Negative thoughts can have very real physical manifestations. So for optimum healing, be careful what you think about and dwell upon.

Experiments which involve the use of placebo medications often demonstrate good examples of the power of the human mind. A recent study at Columbia University tested the effect of belief as it relates to physical reactions and sensations. Participants were administered two instances of skin cream; one batch was said to reduce pain, the other to have no effect on it. The cream was placed on different parts of the subjects' arms, and heat was then applied to the point of causing a burning sensation. The subjects reported that those spots covered with pain-reducing cream felt less of the burning as compared to the areas covered with the neutral cream. Brain scans measuring pain response confirmed their reports.

The applied creams were exactly the same. Translated: what you tell yourself and what you believe may materialize into reality.

During these trying times of injury recovery, it may be difficult to see the bright side of things, day in and day out. You may not always experience high levels of cheer, but be especially careful of letting pessimism consume you. A pessimistic outlook can promote a negative self-image, and among other things, increase your level of stress. Such an undesirable combination can progress to the point where you may feel defeated, helpless, and hopeless in the struggle against your foot condition…which in turn can spawn panic. When you panic, you experience the dramatic "fight or flight" response. This response is your body's inborn reaction to real or imagined threats, one that prepares you to fight back or run away. You would never want to live without the ability to summon the fight or flight response; it can save your life in an emergency. But having it activated regularly for a long period of time can really wear on a person. And it can slow down your recuperation process.

For instance, a by-product of extreme stress such as that caused by the fight or flight response is the hormone cortisol. Among other things, the presence of high cortisol levels can stymie your body's immune response. Cortisol hinders the repair of muscle and connective tissue, making existing injuries more likely to remain so. Therefore, the less cortisol and other nasty by-products of stress you have saturating your tissues, the better your progress will be when healing from plantar fasciitis.

High stress also increases muscle tension. Tension will tighten those muscles up when they should be loose and flexible, helping you move efficiently and protecting you. Tense muscles are more susceptible to strains, tears, and cramps. And in your particular case, those key muscle groups of the lower leg and foot won't operate smoothly, and support for your vulnerable plantar fascia will be reduced. Nobody can lead a completely stress-free existence, but do what you can to avoid stressful scenarios, and relieve stress in ways that work for you. Commit to it.

On a less scientific note, a nasty bout with plantar fasciitis can bring on good old-fashioned discouragement. If you're feeling down and whipped as the condition endures, how likely are you to carry through with efforts needed to heal yourself of plantar fasciitis? Not very. Of course, being optimistic and on top of your game is not always easy. It's tough to see everyone else walking and running all over without a hint of pain, while you can't walk around the block.

Allowed to run rampant, this cloudy sky engulfing your spirit could change your way of living. You might get in the habit of sulking, become sedentary and lethargic, and lead a self-defeating existence. Self-pity, which serves no valuable purpose, could take the place of ambition and activity. Many people lead their whole life without acquiring a condition like plantar fasciitis. Why you?

Well, why not you? Life is full of challenges, and plantar fasciitis just happens to be one you're facing currently. The condition itself is impediment enough; you can't afford any extra negativity. Don't picture yourself as an invalid or a cripple. You're strong, resilient, and capable, but sidelined with a nasty and sadly very prevalent condition. But it's a temporary condition, if you choose to beat it. Whether you spend your present moments in a state of enthusiasm or a state of gloom, the time will go by either way. Decide to be positive, remember the situation won't be around forever, and count on each day being another step toward full recovery.

An important practice recommended to athletes by sports psychologists is the act of positive visualization. The basic concept involves picturing over and over a perfect performance, a flawless execution of the actions, and a successful outcome. The athlete is never to imagine tripping up, or missing a swing, or dropping a ball. Only success. Only the perfect outcome. And with these images of an ideal performance follows the realization of it. Many athletes swear by this visualization-to-reality process. In a similar way, you can picture a successful outcome to your ordeal. See in your mind's eye fully functional, pain-free feet. Even try to feel them. Know with certainty that your feet can return to a stable, healthy state. And in a matter of time, they will. In the high-stakes game of plantar fasciitis recovery, you now know what it takes to win. So carry through on this knowledge, and expect to win.

Don't forget to practice the proper caution and engage in sensible activities, but move on nonetheless. Once you've committed to your recovery plan and stuck with it a while, the routine will become second nature, as will the better choices and better habits. So don't proceed with your day in fear, proceed with confidence. If you go a little too far or do a little too much, ratchet your efforts back a bit. If you make your feet ache now and again by walking or standing more than you should have, know that you haven't canceled out all your good efforts.

Your body is adaptable, and will help you overcome any indiscretions and slight reinjuries you may experience. Just learn from it and adjust.

Plantar fasciitis is an obstacle, and a big one. But people overcome all kinds of obstacles. Don't dwell on the problem to excess. Be confident and patient, do what needs to be done, and you will prevail against plantar fasciitis.

Appendix A: Medical Procedures Related to Plantar Fasciitis

The following is but a brief overview of a few procedures some folks battling with plantar fasciitis choose to undergo. This book does not advocate these treatments, it just describes them. To make an informed decision whether any of them are for you or not, consult a physician.

Corticosteroid Injections

You may be tempted to seek out a quick fix for your condition, and who wouldn't while suffering from plantar fasciitis? That quick fix may appear to you in the form of a corticosteroid injection, which is meant to reduce swelling and pain. The injection often does just that, but its effects are usually temporary. And the temporary relief may come with grave consequences.

The majority of experts agree, corticosteroid injections can come with some nasty side effects. Some of these side effects are as follows:

- Muscle damage in the immediate area.
- Complete rupture of the fascia (as opposed to the much milder micro-tears associated with plantar fasciitis).
- Skin pigmentation changes.
- Injury to peripheral nerves.
- Atrophy of the fat pad in your heel (padding which provides crucial protection).

Repeated injections increase these risks. What's more, the injections are not meant to fix what caused plantar fasciitis in the first place. Use extreme caution before submitting to corticosteroid injections. If you decide to look into corticosteroid injections, you may want to get more than one doctor's opinion.

I personally chose to stick to conservative home care techniques instead. I preferred to address the causes of plantar fasciitis rather than simply delay its symptoms.

Surgery

In general, surgery is not considered as an option until six months of conservative treatment have failed to produce significant results.

And only then, if at all. During surgery for plantar fasciitis part of the plantar fascia will be released, or in other words *cut*, to ease the tension and relieve inflammation.

The easing or releasing of tension on the plantar fascia is of course what the flexibility exercises described earlier in this book are meant to achieve. Stretching may be an easier, safer, and quicker way to accomplish the same goal, with very little chance of negative side effects. In fact, experts agree that surgery is usually not needed to heal a case of plantar fasciitis. Most plantar fasciitis sufferers, about 95%, manage to overcome the condition without surgical treatment.

And surgery provides no guarantees. The New England Journal of Medicine reports that in approximately 25% of all people who have surgery for plantar fasciitis, the heel pain remains.

If you've been struggling with plantar fasciitis for more than six months, and conservative treatment does not seem to do the trick, you may want to discuss surgery as an option with a specialist. But use caution. And make sure to ask about the more modern, less invasive *extracorporeal shockwave therapy*, described next.

Extracorporeal Shockwave Therapy

Extracorporeal shockwave therapy uses ultrasound waves to encourage healing, in the hopes that the waves delivered to the affected area promote the creation of new blood vessels and result in better blood flow. It is also theorized that the brain will better "recognize" the injured area after the stimulation, and then send key nutrients to the location to further expedite healing.

It is a noninvasive procedure, so no cutting will take place. Often an ultrasound image of the foot is taken, and the medical staff determines the greatest area of pain according to your description. Then the treatment is delivered using a device which focuses the waves directly on the injured area.

No anesthesia is necessary to complete extracorporeal shockwave therapy. Nowadays, the entire procedure can be done in the doctor's office in about 10 minutes.

Extracorporeal shockwave therapy has been used now for several years to treat plantar fasciitis, and is considered a low-risk procedure. But like surgery, only a person who has experienced plantar fasciitis for at least six months would be considered for this treatment. It can be quite costly as well.

But remember, conservative, self-directed therapy as described earlier in this book will do things extracorporeal shockwave therapy does not do: fix what ailed you in the first place. After all, if the underlying causes of plantar fasciitis remain, the condition can return regardless of your undergoing this procedure.

Foot Taping

Another noninvasive course of action you might want to consider to protect your injury is foot taping. Like the other items described in this section, a taped foot won't fix what caused plantar fasciitis; but the stability provided by a securely taped foot will prevent additional injury as you stand, walk, and otherwise move about.

In my case, I never used foot taping. I was pretty much "out of the woods" regarding the acute, intensely painful stage of plantar fasciitis by the time I heard how effective foot taping is from a few sources firsthand. To protect my feet in a similar manner, I had already turned to better footwear and over-the-counter inserts. These items were an immense help, so I didn't look further into the foot support side of the equation. Good, protective shoes and in some cases orthotics will often provide the same support and protection that foot taping will, and are much more convenient. In any event, I encourage you to look into foot taping as an option, but have not included a how-to on foot taping in these pages.

All 30 suggestions listed in this book were actions and principles I pretty much lived for a year, and many of them I've incorporated into my daily life. In hindsight, foot taping could have been included among them. Maybe it should be the 31st suggestion in this book. But I don't feel comfortable describing the actual technique of a procedure I've never used myself, especially one which is pretty exact. You don't just cover your foot with tape and call it done. If you feel solid, supportive footwear is still not doing the trick, and you choose to use foot taping, have someone in the sports medicine field show you the correct technique in person. Foot taping could serve as a useful ally during the time you're building up strength and increasing flexibility in your feet and legs. It may allow you to keep moving and working while staving off further injury.

Appendix B: A Celebrity Fitness Author Weighs In

As a reader, you may be pleased to know I got some very helpful input from **Phil Campbell**, author of *Ready, Set, GO! Synergy Fitness*. Phil has trained and guided thousands of athletes and fitness enthusiasts, beginner and advanced alike. His advice has appeared in publications such as *The Los Angeles Times, Self, Outside,* and *O, The Oprah Magazine*, in addition to others. Among other fitness topics, Phil has in-depth knowledge of plantar fasciitis and its causes. Here are some direct recommendations for you, straight from a coach and trainer who's been at it for years:

> "I've worked with over 12,000 athletes and the great majority of them have weak feet due to living life on concrete and wearing cushioned, mini high-heeled sports shoes.
>
> "The wonderful technology of cushioned sports shoes that allows us to live life on hard surfaces has a downside: weak feet, tight Achilles, and extremely tight hamstrings, which show up frequently as plantar problems. The best solution I've found is a twofold strategy: strengthen the shin muscles (anterior tibialis) and ligaments on top of the feet that support the plantar fascia with one set of reverse calf raises to failure once a week, 3x20 reps of calf raises (one set duck-footed, one set pigeon-toed, and one set straight) one time a week, and stretching that targets hamstrings 4 times a week, because tight hamstrings shorten stride length.
>
> "High cushioned heels, which are necessary because we live life on concrete, also keeps the foot from fully dorsiflexing when walking (and running) so the feet don't get a full range of motion and adapt by becoming tight and weak. Since we can't walk barefooted, and wearing flat shoes on concrete may lead to other joint problems like back and knee pain, don't throw away the cushioned sports shoes, but do add the exercises and the stretching to undo what living life on concrete does to us in today's society."

Phil sums it up very succinctly. Common footwear coupled with the unforgiving surfaces of our modern world pose challenges for our foot health. But damage can be undone with the right actions on your part. For more details on the specifics he recommends, visit his website at http://www.readysetgofitness.com/

His book describes not only rehab related to plantar fasciitis, but a whole range of fitness guidance. Check it out!

Appendix C: Recovery Happens

Throughout this book's researching and writing journey, I had the good fortune to talk with a number of people who had traveled a similar road to mine and yours: finding their way through the plantar fasciitis recovery maze. Like us, these folks were pounced upon by the plantar fasciitis beast. And they turned the tables on it.

Let's hear what they had to say.

Gail began with a statement which is oh-so-true: "Just the thought of having plantar fasciitis again is painful!"

Agreed. Very much so. She continued, "Once you've had it, it makes you more aware of your foot health and the way you treat your feet. Mine resulted from multiple sources. I had two ankle surgeries in the mid 1980s and likely developed poor habits in the way I moved my legs and feet while playing sports afterward. Constant pounding on a hard surface such as a tennis court (I used to play a lot of singles) and walking on concrete didn't help matters. I would ice and elevate for a little while and go back at it (physical therapy didn't seem to help at that time)."

Gail found the pain caused by plantar fasciitis was best alleviated with lots of rest and the help of a quality physical therapist. "A new PT revealed that I was walking awkwardly, helped me correct my gait and taught me isolated stretching exercises to do each day. Also, when the excruciating pain of the plantar area occurs, a prescribed walking boot, rest and patience go a long way toward recovery.

"It's disturbing when you feel like you should be conquering the world and this small area of your body relegates you to hobbling like a centenarian. Patience is the key to getting back to just walking, and getting to know how to treat your feet in a healthy way will help avoid plantar fasciitis in the future."

Gail follows through on her philosophy with action.

"I still stretch, and it's been about three years since I was told I had plantar fasciitis...foot, heel, calf: everything that's connected. I stretch a bit before I get out of bed, random times during the day and before and after a workout. I find that even at my 'tender young age' of 43, I have to stretch most all muscles in my body before I get out of bed or they don't work as fluidly as I'd like."

She then added her thoughts regarding a well-known plantar fasciitis victim.

"The next time Shaquille O'Neill sits out a game because of what you think is a minor foot injury, think again. Cheer for his speedy recovery as much as you do his next dunk!"

Well said, Gail!

Key points: Avoid brutal surfaces. Once you do recover, respect your body even more and remember the types of things that cause plantar fasciitis in the first place. Use an ideal foot strike when you walk and run. Value rest. Be patient. And make sure to stretch both when in recovery, and as a preventive measure even after you are healed up.

Tim is a runner, and became one of countless runners to hit the plantar fasciitis wall.

"Like many runners, I had a bad case of plantar fasciitis in both feet," Tim said. "I would wake up in the morning and literally hobble across the room to turn off the alarm clock. It was so painful even to walk in the morning before my feet loosened up a bit."

He overcame the initial hurdle with a solid pair of shoe inserts. "As soon as I started using Superfeet insoles in my running shoes, nearly all my foot problems went away. I have no connection with the company (don't even know who makes them!) other than being a satisfied customer. They really were lifesavers!"

But like other savvy former sufferers of the dreaded foot condition, he didn't let down his guard. He continued to address factors that can cause plantar fasciitis in the first place.

"Stretching is key," said Tim. "I've found, actually, that stretching AFTER running helps more than anything. I used to just walk home after finishing my run, and that was my entire 'cool down.' I've since found that stretching calves, ankles, and arches even just for a minute or so upon arriving at home seems to make a huge difference in recovery and eliminating stiffness or pain.

"I also try to loosen my ankles and arches a couple of times a day, just sitting in my office; I'll bend, stretch and roll my feet around to get everything feeling loose and get the blood flowing. I keep a little mini soccer ball under my desk as well, just to have something slightly different for my feet to rest on or fidget with throughout the day. I don't have any doctor's advice to back this up, but my feet and ankles just seem to feel better if I can keep them loose and active throughout the day rather than trying to really loosen them only before a run or workout."

Key points: Good footwear, including a proven insert, can make a huge difference. He is staying active, and maintaining flexibility, blood flow, and strength in his feet. Even if new footwear improves your situation, stay on task, and keep the momentum working in your favor. Strengthen, stretch, exercise, and protect yourself from the injury's recurrence. And keep plantar fasciitis at bay for good.

Author's note: like Tim, I too have used Superfeet brand inserts with success. And like Tim, I have zero affiliation with the company. I will say I found Superfeet to be one of several great inserts out on the market; consider using a pair.

Barbara experienced the plantar fasciitis onslaught from an all-too-common cause – working on her feet for hours at a time, while on that culprit that invades most of our lives: an unyielding surface. Here was her experience:

"I'm a nurse. Hence many hours of walking, walking, and more walking on hard linoleum floors. After years and years of this, I developed plantar fasciitis. At the end, just before leaving my hospital job, my feet were on fire within 10 minutes of starting my shift."

Ouch. I can just feel it. Bad memories.

She continued, "So I left that job/profession and went overseas to teach English (!). Instead, I found a privately-owned health clinic which hired me as their nurse manager (lots of sitting and a small facility, so minimal walking). Buoyed by this experience, I went to another clinic job (actually an embassy health unit). Again, lots of sitting with a tiny bit of walking around (on a carpeted floor). I was there for 2 years. I also limited my outside-of-work walking - took buses, trams, etc. whenever possible. And I always found a place to sit, no standing around for this girl.

"After about 3 years of this regimen, I realized my feet felt better. It's been a couple of years now and my plantar fasciitis doesn't bother me at all. However, I still sit rather than stand, ride my bike rather than walk, and if I do walk too much, my feet feel pretty tired afterwards. I think I could relapse easily.

"I might mention that I visited a podiatrist, tried shoe inserts, strapping (horrible!), stretching exercises and of course, ibuprofen. None of that worked for me. My recommendation is 'get off your feet.'"

Key points: There is no substitute for rest. A person must find a way to avoid the factors which brought on the plantar fasciitis condition. If this is not done, the condition will often worsen. Sometimes, a new way of living must be embraced to do this; in some cases, this could mean a different line or style of work, as Barbara found.

Author's note: Stretching and strengthening will almost always help, and never hurt, when on the plantar fasciitis road to recovery. However, if injurious activity continues to take place, the benefits of those rehab efforts can be minimized. The sooner stretching and strengthening are put to use, the better. And that goes double for putting a halt to the factors which are aggravating the condition in the first place.

And finally:

Randy has a tale that, if you feel hopeless and overwhelmed by your foot injury, might make you take pause. Your foot injury situation, although never pleasant, may be less complicated than it sometimes seems when taken in perspective. As told by Randy, a 6-year cancer survivor and plantar fasciitis victim for over 3 years:

"I had worn thin little loafer type shoes for years at my job, but resigned when pregnant with the triplets…in other words, I had not worn good arch support as a rule. When my triplets were 14 months old, a routine mammogram showed early breast cancer. I had a mastectomy and chemo. All was well and I did not do reconstruction at the time due to the longer recovery needed. I always said I'd have reconstruction when they went to school and I had time for a longer recovery. Fast forward just one year after that surgery.

"I did three days worth of 'hard on my feet' tasks (walking at an amusement park, standing on a hard tile floor for hours, doing projects, house cleaning). When I woke up the next day, I couldn't walk. My feet felt swollen and I was in pain. As time went on, I realized I limped from the bed to the bathroom each morning, every time I got up from a seated position, and especially had trouble when I got out of a car and walked toward my destination. I tried to hide how much annoying and chronic pain I was in. My hip then ended up with bursitis from me 'walking funny' for so long due to my foot pain."

Over 3 years plus, Randy went to two podiatrists, a chiropractor, and an orthopedist. She wore a night splint, took anti-inflammatory and pain medication, and wore custom inserts. She rolled an iced bottle as well as a tennis ball under her feet. Still the heel pain remained.

She even turned to "excruciating shots of cortisone," as she described them, which turned out to be ineffective. No surprise there.

"I was resigned that, though I'd beat cancer, I was going to have to live with this forever...like walking on a sprained ankle all the time! I didn't remember what 'normal' felt like anymore. I tried not to talk about it or whine or complain...who wants to hear that? And it surely didn't help! But I was in chronic pain!" she said.

Then came the breakthrough.

"I scheduled my breast reconstruction when the triplets were in kindergarten," Randy continued. "Due to a family history of heart issues and my age, the doctor wanted heart clearance before surgery: a full stress test and such. (All results were normal, but that wasn't the best part!) The 15 minutes or less I spent on the slowly elevating treadmill, walking faster and faster, stretched my fascia gradually (I deduce) and that night I realized, I was in a lot less pain. The next morning, I got out of bed and walked without my characteristic slow limp. I could not believe, after everything I'd done to solve my plantar fasciitis, that those 15 minutes CURED it! This was 1 1/2 years ago and I have not had ONE bout of foot/arch/heel pain since!"

She adds that her story, "…was long and involved, but truly, to have this "benefit" of my breast cancer (in a roundabout way) was SUCH a blessing!"

She sounds excited, and who in her shoes wouldn't? Over 3 years of pain with each step she took, staving off cancer, and triplets to take care of! Randy's ordeal just goes to show, you don't know when the tides may turn in your favor, and what extra ingredient may complete the perfect recipe for plantar fasciitis recovery.

> **Key points**: Active recovery is more often than not a key contributor to healing a case of plantar fasciitis. And stretching is crucial. In this case, the Achilles tendon and calf area became more flexible through high-motion exercise on a treadmill. For other people, that flexibility is best developed through a more controlled method, like slow, gentle stretching. In any case, flexibility needs to be introduced to take tension off the fascia and allow it to heal.

> Author's note: Did Randy's use of foot massage through the iced bottle and tennis ball help in any way? And did her upgrade in footwear? Most likely a yes to both…it's possible those actions were just not enough by themselves. She eventually found that final key to put the odds in her favor, and allow the healing to commence.

As these success stories illustrate, plantar fasciitis is often healed through a combination of actions and factors. Have faith in yourself and your ability to heal. Once again, make that commitment to rid yourself of the condition. And find that individualized, magic combination that solves the puzzle of your own plantar fasciitis recovery. It'll happen.

Index

About the Author

Patrick Hafner has been involved in fitness and conditioning for over 30 years. He competed for 15 years in wrestling sports, winning numerous state, regional, and international titles, and has worked as a strength training adviser and judo instructor. As a hiking enthusiast, Patrick has explored trails all over North America and Europe. As a runner, he has completed over 70 races. Patrick holds a B.S. in Kinesiology from the University of Minnesota.

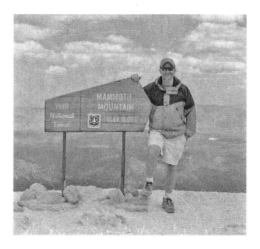

CPSIA information can be obtained at www.ICGtesting.com
Printed in the USA
BVOW071629110912

300150BV00002B/164/P

9 780980 172454